The Girl Who Swallowed Office Supplies

Stories from the Life of a Mental Health Social Worker

Belinda Sutton Mitchell

Dedication

To my children, who put up with this social worker when she was strung out, stressed out, and at times overwhelmed by her chosen work. Thank you for your love, understanding, and cutting me slack when I needed it but didn't deserve it.

To social workers and caregivers of the intellectually challenged and/or mentally ill, who are overworked, underpaid, and undervalued. Even without rewards and recognition you show up. Thank you for all you do.

To Damian, Cara, Jesse, Sereadia, and (former) Officer Nick.

There is a quote that has been attributed to Margaret Mead: "Never doubt that a small group of thoughtful, committed citizens can change the world. Indeed, it is the only thing that ever has."

You changed the life, the world, of one small girl with Down syndrome when social services looked away. I am honored to know you.

Acknowledgments

This being my first book, I had fear and trepidation during the entire writing process. Numerous "cheerleaders" encouraged me: friends, family, co-workers. I can't begin to name them all. But a special thanks goes to Gary Kerr and Tack Chumbley who spent so much time making suggestions and "cleaning up" my manuscript, and to my son Andrew for trying to make me more photogenic!

Sarah Mitchell designed my book cover, and my wonderful team through fivrr. pulled it all together. I am truly blessed.

Prologue

I am a social worker.

I didn't plan to become a social worker. My interest was in political science and foreign languages. But somewhere along the line I realized I didn't want to be in politics, and I have no gift for foreign languages. When it was time to declare a major at the University of Alabama, I was stumped. After discarding various suggestions made by friends, I picked up the college course catalog and perused the subjects in various schools. I selected social work simply by default. No noble purpose, just trying to evade higher mathematics.

Fast forward. I became a real, honest-to-goodness social worker. But there was one thing I didn't realize until it was too late. Although I loved the daily field work, I discovered I would never be well off financially. No educational counselor ever told us that. I guess if we knew what we would earn when we graduated, most of us would have changed majors. But it didn't really matter at that point. I had fallen in love with the work itself.

And instead of banking money through the years for my retirement and travel, I banked stories. I collected them in old journals, on the back of used envelopes, in wide-ruled, spiral-bound notebooks and on legal pads. I jotted down notes on the backs of bank deposit slips, index cards, napkins, and on hundreds and hundreds of post-it notes.

Every story I have written about actually happened. Others may remember certain details differently; in my family, we sometimes remember events in ways that conflict with each other, even though we were all present. I have written what I personally recall, using quotation marks and dialogue to make my stories more readable.

At times I have included my opinions and observations. I have changed names, ages, locations, and even chronology in order to protect the privacy of those involved. I have not recorded these stories to embarrass or vilify anyone but to shine a small light into the life of the mentally ill, as well as the challenges of those who care for them. Every person I have written was/is a real person. Every single incident I wrote about is true. I know. I was there.

My name is Belinda, and I am a social worker. These are some of my stories.

Contents

CHAPTER 1

Learning Curve

Old Mr. Sampson had a somewhat addled wife, but he was as cunning as he was funny and engaging. He tried, and failed, to wheedle me into falsifying an application to receive additional government funding to which he was not entitled. Afterwards, he pouted a bit, but we soon became friends.

On the other hand, there was Mr. Hallman. Although I visited with him many times, I think he barely tolerated my company. Perhaps he saw me for what I was: a naive woman, young enough to be his granddaughter, who presented herself to him as someone who could "help." These two men were my first clients.

Mr. Hallman was a tall, angular man in his early seventies who stood straight-backed, head erect, with a no-nonsense expression on his face. My supervisor told me prior to our first visit that he had just been released from prison after serving thirty years. I was assigned to visit and determine what he needed. When I knocked on the front door of his housing project apartment, I was directed to one of two straight-backed wooden chairs on the front porch. After introducing myself, I tried to make casual conversation but received only short, curt answers interspersed with awkward silences. I soon ran out of topics to break the ice. So, I blurted out the question that I had been holding in since I arrived.

"Mr. Hallman, I hear you just got out of prison. What did you do?"

"Shot and killed my wife."

"Oh." His face was expressionless, and he was staring out across the yard.

Silence.

I waited, shifting in my chair a bit.

"Well," I finally said. "You were in prison a long time, plenty of time to think about what you did. I'm sure if you could go back, you would handle things differently."

He continued to stare out across the yard.

"No," he said, calmly and deliberately. "I would shoot her again."

He paused as I sat there, stunned at what I had just heard. Then he continued in a flat, unemotional voice.

"I caught her in bed with my best friend."

"Oh," was all I could reply.

First lesson learned: don't patronize. Ask questions and think before you spout off.

I had to be embarrassed a second time before I actually learned the lesson. Visiting a sweet, elderly lady in another unit of the same housing project, I noticed the cozy touches around the room: a round lace doily on a small table, a rocking chair, family pictures on the wall. Suddenly, we heard a loud "pop" outside the apartment. She looked startled. I slipped easily into my "helper" mode.

"It's all right," I said calmly, as if trying to soothe a young child. "I'm sure that was a car back firing. Nothing to be alarmed about."

She sat straighter in her chair. "No, dear," she said firmly. "*That* was a gun shot."

I walked to the window and looked out. People were starting to gather, and soon we heard a siren and two police officers drove up in a patrol car.

She was right. It *was* a gunshot. Two men had an altercation across the street, and one shot the other one in the front yard. Dead.

In the early years I taught a class of intellectually challenged adults. They worked on life skills, like learning their addresses and phone numbers. They learned how to call 911 in an emergency. They practiced basic hygiene and oral care. They traced letters until they could write their names. Some had the capability not only to learn but to retain information. For some, it wasn't within their ability. They would work all week, and on Friday they could show me what they learned. But when they returned on Monday, the knowledge was gone. And we would start again.

I gave a lot of thought to how to make my classroom a better learning environment. Since there was repetition involved, I wanted to make it as interesting as possible. One of my ideas was to bring a hamster into the classroom. The students could take turns feeding it, learning how to care for a pet.

Everyone loved our new addition. Well, almost everyone.

Randy was a tall, scrawny, dark-haired boy who rarely smiled. His hair was long, greasy, and unkempt. I guessed from his well-worn, ill-fitting clothes that his family struggled to get by. He was one of the highest functioning students in my class and seemed eager to learn about most things. But not about hamsters.

Randy's turn came, and I reminded him that the hamster needed to be fed. He looked startled and began backing away, shaking his head. He didn't say a word but continued to slowly shake his head as he backed into a corner of the room, far away from the hamster cage. I didn't understand. Although shy, he usually was involved and cooperative.

"Randy? It's your turn to feed the hamster. He won't hurt you."

He was silent but continued to shake his head.

"Randy, this is your responsibility. Please feed him," I insisted. "He's hungry."

Suddenly tears welled up in Randy's eyes. In a soft, almost imperceptible voice he whispered, "I can't. Please don't make me. I can't."

The entire class had been observing our interaction. Realizing there was more to this than defiance, I turned the students' attention to handwork on the table in front of them before approaching Randy. He was still standing in the corner, slightly trembling.

"Randy," I said quietly.

"What's wrong?"

Big tears spilled down his cheeks. "I can't get close to it," he finally got out. "I don't like him."

"Why?" I asked. "Are you afraid of him?"

He sniffled. "He looks like a rat."

"And you don't like rats?"

"No." The tears were flowing now, dripping from his chin onto the floor. "They crawl on me when I'm asleep and bite me on the face.

My eyes opened wide in horror. "That's awful! You don't have to do anything with that hamster. The others will take care of him."

He wiped his tears away and tried to smile, and though he couldn't seem to get it out, I saw gratitude in his eyes.

We talked a lot about hygiene in our daily classes: the importance of bathing, wearing clean clothes, washing hair, brushing teeth. One large young man stood out because of his body odor. He was friendly and eager to please, but some days it was hard to be around him, especially in the summertime. We had discussed bathing until I was tired of bringing up the topic. One day I pulled him aside to have a private pep talk.

"James," I began, "you know we have talked about taking a shower every day."

"Yes ma'am," he said.

"I don't think you are doing that. Is there a problem?"

He hung his head, embarrassed. "Well," he said. "I don't got no soap at my house."

"Why don't I bring you some soap tomorrow, and when you get home you can take a shower. How's that?"

He looked down at the floor. "Well," he said slowly, "sometime we don't got no water either." Then he raised his head tentatively, "But sometime we *do*."

I thought about this. "Okay, James. I will bring you soap to take home. And whenever you have water, take a shower. Will that work for you?"

He grinned slightly. "Yes ma'am. That will work."

James and Randy taught me a lot early in my social work career. Don't assume everyone is like you. Don't assume they have food in their homes or sleep on a mattress. Don't assume their space is clean, safe, or inviting. Don't assume they have a can opener to open a can of soup, or a stove that works with which to boil an egg. Don't assume they are cared for at home. Don't even assume they have a home. Don't assume they have access to a pencil, or a piece of paper. Don't assume anything. Listen, and watch for cues. There is always a reason behind the behavior. Try to find it.

CHAPTER 2

Mental Illness

I am curious by nature, fascinated by what makes people tick. My experience with those who have mental disorders has been over many years, but I do not claim to be an expert. That is, unless you use the definition of an expert to be someone who knows enough in a specific field to realize how much they *don't* know. I *don't* know a lot.

I have never been interested in supervising others and didn't seek a post-graduate degree. I wanted to problem solve and work directly with my clients. I wanted to make a difference. Sometimes I think I have succeeded; other times I know I have failed. But I keep trying.

People with mental illnesses are not much different than us. In fact, they *are* us. The National Alliance on Mental Illness (NAMI) says that in any given year, one in five adults experience mental illness and one in twenty adults experience a serious mental illness that substantially interferes with or limits major life activities. The stats are similar for children ages six to seventeen. One in six experiences a mental health disorder each year, with only about half receiving treatment. Perhaps these numbers help explain NAMI's motto: "You are not alone."

Each of us is on a health continuum, whether physical or mental. No one is 100 percent whole in either category. And while some mental illnesses have specific criteria to diagnose them, others are less absolute, at least as far as most of us are concerned. Whether we are willing to admit it or not, we all have our idiosyncrasies. For example, you may insist on having your clothing folded or organized in a specific way. You call yourself a perfectionist. But think carefully Do you *like* your clothes that way? Or do you *need* them that way to not feel anxious? Do you feel driven to do something (like fold clothes or wash hands) repetitively? Does it interfere with your life activities? Then you start leaning toward what professionals call *obsessive-compulsive disorder* (OCD).

Sadness is a normal emotion. Sometimes our sadness may be so deep and prolonged that it adversely affects our ability to function. Is it still sadness? Or have we moved to depression? Is it mild, or do we meet the criteria for clinical depression and need treatment?

What about fear? Paranoia? Anxiety?

The more extreme we get in our behavior, the more dysfunctional we become and the more likely we are to meet the criteria for true mental illness.

In my parents' generation, mental illness wasn't discussed in public settings. It was as if it didn't exist. But most families had someone in them who was considered strange or eccentric. They were usually described as "odd." Some old movies used the word "pixelated" to describe these behavioral quirks.

I had a dear, elderly relative who heard things. Any noise she heard in her attic was attributed to the "Russians who live up there." When she left her house, she would sometimes leave notes for the "people who lived in the TV." She was convinced that Dan Rather was sending her private messages during the CBS Evening News. She believed they had a standing date each weeknight night at 5:30 pm, and he was flirting with her through the television screen. Once she even claimed he tried to look up her dress. Sadly, she lived for years with her delusions, few people being aware of her psychoses. It didn't occur to the family to have her mental health checked out by a psychiatrist. She was no danger to herself or others. Most of the time, she worked a full-time job, regularly attended church, and was well thought of by her neighbors and coworkers. I suspect she herself knew something was off but learned to hide it from others. I remember her as a sweet, caring person who loved dogs and babies. In her later years she seemed confused and anxious.

Mental illness has always carried with it a stigma that only now is beginning to lessen. Social media has sped this process along. What people could never say out loud to a friend or coworker, they now post online for everyone to see. It's as if they feel anonymous over the Internet and somehow less vulnerable. But they feel the need to get it out there. That is a good thing, because if a mental disorder is hidden it cannot be addressed and treated.

I have dealt with all types of people and all types of disorders. I have worked with individuals and families with problems in almost every area imaginable: domestic assault, sexual abuse, depression, stalking, gambling addiction, anxiety, phobias. I have worked with people with borderline personality disorder, schizophrenia, and bipolar disorder, as well as disorders that are not as well known. I am much too familiar with narcissistic personality disorder. On the happier side of social work, I have assisted families with adoption, and I loved being part of life-changing child placements. But the bulk of my work has been in the mental health field.

The hardest clients for me to work with are those who are either borderline or mildly intellectually challenged. They struggle between two worlds: that of the "normal" person and the world of those who can do little on their own due to lack of ability. That is not to say they cannot achieve, but they need a support system and cannot do it independently.

They know they are not like everyone else, but they hope against hope that they can someday be "normal," just ordinary, and fit into the communities around them. I can't imagine the pain they must feel, being on the very edge of society and yet never quite fitting in.

I remember a scrawny teenager named Ronald, from many years ago. He was what we used to call borderline mentally retarded (MR), a slow learner. If he had been given extra attention and the advantages of growing up in a solid, middle-class, "average" family with its privileges, I think his future would have looked much different. But his family was dirt poor, dysfunctional and struggled for daily necessities, including clean water. His house, located in a high crime area, was infiltrated with rats. Each day was focused on survival. Ronald might or might not get to school. He might or might not have clean clothes to wear, or water to bathe in, or food for lunch. The family struggled to survive; there was no time, energy, or resources to focus on Ronald's needs. And so, he slipped farther and farther back in school, retreating from those around him. He was mocked by some of his classmates for poor hygiene and smelling bad. He wasn't as quick as the other kids, so they called him a "retard." And that is how he came to view himself. By the time he came on my radar, his self-esteem was so low you couldn't find it.

But his eyes . . . That was over twenty-five years ago, and I still remember his wistful eyes. Ronald didn't want to be rich, or a movie star, or travel to far-off places. He just wanted to not be different, to escape people's attention. He wanted a job at McDonald's, a decent place to live, and friends who wouldn't make fun of him. Life had pushed him down so many times that the longing to be normal was all that was left. He had no hope, just an acceptance of his unchanging life.

It made me sad. And angry. Why are some of us born into families full of love, hope, and stability yet others are born into nothing but despair? I didn't have to grow up with the challenges Ronald grew up with. Why was I special?

But I knew the answer. I am not special. Some things just happen.

I am still grieved that Ronald suffered so much. I was sad that there are many others like him, and I was angry that I could not change his life. I sometimes feel guilty that my life has had so many advantages over his, especially as I was growing up.

My mother was a homemaker, and my father was a rural preacher who farmed on a small scale. My mother's grandfather was, among other things, a worm farmer. My grandfather on my dad's side was a white sharecropper who grew cotton in north Alabama. I was the first person in my large, extended family to finish college. There was never enough money in our family, but we didn't consider ourselves poor. We were just short on money.

We knew what it was like to do without. But we always had clean clothes, a warm bed, and plenty of food, much of which we grew ourselves. We had books, lots of books. We were taught never to look down on someone who had less than we did and to share what we had. There was lots of hard work, love, and laughter in our house.

After college I married and followed my husband's career from state to state, city to city. We lived in big cities and small towns. In the process, I associated mostly with people who were at least relatively affluent and some who were quite wealthy. I no longer was around people who had their water or power cut off because they couldn't pay. Our conversations were not about where groceries were the cheapest or what days the thrift store put out its best merchandise. We talked about travel, theater, politics. We talked about good books, concerts, and our visions for the future. Slowly, I left behind the world of payday loans and Dollar General. The problem was not with my friends, or what we talked about or focused on. The problem was that I forgot. I forgot how most people in the world live. I forgot that they didn't live the life I lived; they didn't have the resources, or the opportunities, or the support system I had. They didn't have the privileges.

After my older children left home and the youngest were in their teens, I went back to work in my chosen field. Then I remembered. My service grew, my gratitude grew, and my faith grew. I needed my clients. They helped keep me grounded. They changed me.

CHAPTER 3

Toy Soldier Commander

In the world of the developmentally and intellectually disabled, vocabulary is important. Acceptable terminology changes from generation to generation, decade to decade, and sometimes even year to year. Descriptive words are taken over by popular culture and used as insults. Terms originally used merely as medical definitions, developed by psychologists and other clinicians, became over time insulting and offensive. They were replaced by other words that, over time, became insulting and offensive. The medical diagnosis mental retardation was first changed to MR and then, in 2013, was finally dropped from the DSM-5, the official diagnostic manual of the American Psychiatric Association. It was replaced by "intellectual disability (intellectual developmental disorder)." But already I have begun observing that we are on the road to having to change our terminology again.

Keenan pointed this out to me very clearly several years ago. A young man with moderate intellectual disability (IQ 35–55), he was quite sensitive to how he was labeled. This has become a real challenge for those of us who, from time to time, need to provide descriptions of those with whom we work to identify services and provide needed supports.

I had just completed a state training that included the use of descriptive terminology. There were many "don'ts": don't use the term "patient," don't use the term "disabled," don't use the term "client." OK. But here's the catch: there *was* no correct terminology. The training provided not a single word to use that would be appropriate. When questioned, the trainer simply said he didn't know. Others in the class offered the term "individual," which was unacceptable to me. It was nondescriptive.

Sometimes, we need both adjectives and nouns to identify groups or persons. We are Americans, mothers, cancer survivors, soldiers, students, teachers. We are black, white, redheaded, long legged, curly haired, back country, sophisticated. We are rural, urban. We are described not only by who we are individually but what groups we belong to. In a broad sense they define us. Terms like *addicts* or *enablers* give us a greater understanding of those around us, although we aspire to keep the terms descriptive and not pejorative. And while we are all much more than the groups or categories we belong to, identifying by use of descriptive words assists us to interact with each other on a more humane, personal level.

But I needed a word, so I used the word "individual." Keenan overheard me one day tell someone that he was "an individual that I supported."

"I AM NOT AN INDIVIDUAL," he yelled from the next room. "DON'T SAY THAT WORD!"

Keenan was smart enough to realize that regardless of the word, the definition in context was the same. He had an intellectual disability. After that, for lack of a better term, I began calling those with intellectual disabilities that I worked with, "clients." I explained to them that I was working *for* them, providing a service, which is what attorneys do. So far, so good. I haven't offended anyone as far as I know. But one day I may, and I will have to find another word.

Like many of my younger clients, especially the males in their twenties, Keenan could be physically aggressive at times. He had not one but two designated staff to supervise him, keeping himself and those around him safe. He had recently gone through a particularly rough period with lots of physical aggression, including property damage, and I needed to address the problem at one of my house visits.

Keenan collected green and brown plastic army men. He adored them. He probably had thousands and kept them in large black trash bags in his room. If he had a dollar in his pocket, he would pester staff to take him to Dollar Tree, or Dollar General, or Walmart to buy a small bag of army men to add to his collection. On the day I arrived, the living room was covered with them, and he was deeply involved in play. Staff had helped him turn cardboard boxes into garages for his jeeps and other small army vehicles, and they lined the room. Keenan had organized his army men into units and was moving them around as he gave orders.

I had an epiphany. Maybe I could enter the game and use the plastic army men to make my point. Keenan was a talker and not good at listening, even on his best days; his recent behavior would ultimately send him back to mental health court for accountability and direction. Keenan was not a fan of the judge, even though he often doled out Subway gift cards to those who showed up in his courtroom with good behavior reports.

I made small talk for a few minutes but was mostly ignored. Moving close to the coffee table, I lined up 150 of his toy soldiers. I wanted to make a point using an example of another client who had recently been in mental health court and was sent to jail for five months. Five months equals 150 days. Each plastic soldier represented one day.

“Hey, Keenan,” I said, “look at this. One hundred fifty men are lined up. Each one stands for one day in jail. That’s how long Joey had to stay there because he was fighting and acting out. You need to be on your best behavior. Your soldiers want you to stay out of trouble so the judge won't send you there too."

Keenan glanced over at me, then began removing the soldiers off the coffee table. He took his troops across the room and refused to talk to me anymore that day. The visit was over.

A few weeks later we had a team meeting to discuss what we could do about Keenan's ongoing behavioral issues. He was present and sat quietly for a while, listening. But he kept staring at me from the end of the long conference table. Then he spoke up.

"Miss Belinda," he said with a scowl on his face, "my soldiers told me they don't like you, and they don't want you to touch them anymore. You are not their leader. I am."

Keenan had a roommate who was much higher functioning than he was. Trey had lived at home for a long time before moving in with Keenan and had been spoiled. When his mother could no longer handle him, the state took over. He was arrogant, lazy, and didn't take direction well. He was racist and liked to watch porn. He considered himself superior to both his roommate and staff and felt entitled. He also figured out quickly how to push buttons—those of his staff and especially Keenan's. I try to stay out of roommate squabbles; part of normal development is learning how to resolve interpersonal conflicts and my rescue interference could slow down that process. Unless someone was being physically abused, they were encouraged to work out their differences between themselves.

But one day I walked in and heard Trey calling Keenan names. Keenan was upset and bellowing back.

"I AM NOT A RETARD! I AM NOT A N****R!"

Keenan was about to punch Trey, and I couldn't say I blamed him. I was furious. I broke my rule and raised my voice. "Stop it, Trey. Stop it immediately!"

I let Trey know quite plainly that he could NOT call his roommate a retard or any other name. No racial slurs. He smirked. No apology, just a smirk.

I have worked with hundreds of intellectually challenged clients through the years, and while I had a closer bond with some than others, I had never met one that I didn't like. Until now.

As I processed this new revelation, I felt guilty. Trey had an intellectual disability that he couldn't control. How could I not like him? What was wrong with me? Maybe he needed to be assigned another caseworker. I talked to my supervisor.

"What don't you like about him?" She asked.

"He's arrogant, mean, racist, and thinks he's better than anyone else. He's a jerk."

She smiled slightly, a little amused. “Well, there’s your answer. There’s nothing wrong with you. He’s just not likable.”

As of this writing, I have only come across one other person with limited intellectual ability whom I didn’t like. But this time I didn’t feel guilty. I worked with him one-on-one for several months and concluded that he had all the traits of an undiagnosed psychopath. He just wasn’t likable.

CHAPTER 4

God Don't Like Ugly

John has been a favorite of mine from the first time I met him. He is big. Really big. At 6' 4" and almost 300 pounds, he makes an imposing figure. But inside that twenty-five-year-old body is the mind and emotions of a ten-year-old boy.

John was born intellectually challenged and was eventually diagnosed as bipolar with attention deficit/ hyperactivity disorder (ADHD) and impulse control disorder. When he became anxious, his right arm began to twitch, and he rolled his shoulder upward and back. He explained this as Tourette syndrome from a diagnosis long ago, although I have never seen that documented. And even on his best days, what John said was rarely reliable.

When I first met John, he was eighteen and had recently aged out of the foster care system. I went to visit him at the home he shared with a roommate and staff and introduced myself as his new caseworker. He was wary, stayed away, and watched me from across the room. I knew he was uncomfortable and ignored him until he was ready to talk. After a few minutes he approached the table where I was sitting.

"Hi, John," I said. "My name is Belinda. So glad to meet you."

He stared at me for a moment, then spoke.

"I want you to know something," he said gruffly. "I am not retarded. I know my chart says I am, but I want you to know I am not. So don't call me that."

"I'm glad you told me," I said. "I promise I will never call you retarded."

His shoulder twitched.

"Another thing. I don't want to talk about my family."

"Okay. No family talk unless you want to."

Over the next several visits, John warmed to me and started talking. At first, I was stunned at some of the things he told me. Awful, terrible things. But over time I realized that much of what John said just wasn't true. Some of it was exaggeration, some was truly what he thought he remembered, and some of it was dramatic fantasy made up to impress the listener.

John told me his dad was a metro vice cop gone bad. Not true.

He told me his folks used to lock him in the closet when he was young. True.

He said his mom threw hot spaghetti on him. Maybe.

He said he used to go hungry because they wouldn't feed him. True.

He said his mom died. Not true.

He said his dad was in prison. Not true.

He told me he punched his father in the face and broke his nose because he was being mistreated. True.

He said he lived in Ghana for six months with a foster father. Not true. But he did go on a month-long visit with him. That's when he learned to love African food.

John fabricated detailed stories. This made it difficult for anyone who worked with him to fully understand a situation and respond appropriately. He had a sweet, abused heart underneath all the bluster and aggression. He simply coped the only way he knew how, by telling stories to be the center of attention and using his size to intimidate. He says he learned that from his dad.

As our relationship developed and John learned to trust me, he began sharing a few things. I love my mom and dad he would say, but they mistreated me. I understand, I would tell him. But they are your family. You can still love your mom and dad and know they were terrible parents. They should have protected you, fed you, taken care of you. There is no excuse for how you were treated. But you can still love them. That's okay.

He looked relieved.

John was referred to mental health court for assault on his roommate. The judge was comfortable working with people like John who had severe behavioral problems along with mental disabilities. He approached him with a combination of good judge/bad judge. John made biweekly trips to the court so the judge could keep up with his progress. Depending on the visit, the judge would either scold and threaten jail time or reward him with a Subway gift card for progress made on his behavior problems. I never ceased to be amazed at how John—and others like him—would work so hard for two weeks for a $5.00 Sub sandwich. It was a reminder of the fact that they were intellectually and developmentally challenged, regardless of their size or age. Still, after a time, even gift cards didn't work. At one point I got so frustrated with his behavior that I printed out an online photo of the judge and taped it to his refrigerator, where I knew he would see it twenty times a day. "There," I told John. "There is your reminder to behave." He frowned. But it helped, at least temporarily.

John has always been a handful. Over a ten-year period he blew through six provider agencies. Provider agencies are licensed and responsible for the care of the intellectually challenged people they are assigned by the state. They hire staff, rent homes, and oversee the health, safety, and all activities involved in daily living of those they support. John stayed an average of twenty months with each one before they discharged him. I can truly say that each agency tried to support him in ways that assisted him to become more independent and increase his quality of life. But for day-to-day staff, life with John was incredibly difficult.

One caregiver stood out. Ron was a large man, a little taller than John. He was cool and hip and John called him "Bro." Ron was the stabilizing influence in John's life for many years. They lived together for a few years at a time; then John would blow up and end up in jail, or a psych ward, or both. After he was discharged, John would be moved somewhere else, giving Ron a chance to recover from burnout. But then the new caregiver would become mentally exhausted, and John would go back to live with Ron. Ron understood John as well as anyone could. John once told him that his father abused his mom and that she in turn abused him. He noticed that no matter how overbearing and controlling his father was, she would always take him back. John believed that if he was in control like his father, he would also be accepted back, regardless of what he did. But when he couldn't control everything and everyone, he had to run away or become abusive. He tried to avoid accountability. His father never had to be accountable, why should he? He was simply imitating his father, thinking this was the way to get attention and acceptance. John had precious insight for one so mentally challenged.

Provider agencies who contract with the state to provide services for clients like John not only take on a lot of responsibility, but they also take on a lot of risk to both lives and property. John had been out of control for some time. He had no conservator to help make decisions for him, and as a result, he made lots of poor ones, including, at times, refusing to bathe, refusing to participate in helpful programs, refusing to take his medications, and threatening (and sometimes following through) when he didn't get his way. He had few consequences.

John needed a conservator to help him learn to reign in his behavior, but the state wouldn't pay for it. It was short-sighted on their part, because in addition to John's behavioral problems that caused staff turnover, taxpayers had to fund his many police calls, incarcerations, court appearances, extra staff and much more. The state also spent a lot of money for behavior respites, behavior analysts, and other support personnel. But with clients like John the results were usually minimal. They needed consequences through "tough love" and to be held accountable.

John had a pattern of risky behavior. He made hundreds of police calls over a ten-year period to have himself admitted to psych wards because he "needed a break" from his caregiver. There were a few arrests for assault. The cycle needed to be stopped, but someone had to have some authority over John to make it happen. Since I was no longer his case worker, I figured it might as well be me. So, I found a pro bono attorney, went to court, and due to my experience and relationship with John, was granted conservatorship. It was during a calm week in John's life, and when the judge asked him if he agreed to the arrangement, he said yes.

The first step in fostering independence and self-worth is to focus on personal responsibility and accountability. John and I had a long talk, and I explained that he would have the chance to make his own decisions. But if he chose poorly, like refusing to take his medication or bathe, then I would step in and overrule him. There would be negative consequences for poor choices and rewards for good ones. Some would be natural and some I would impose.

For example, if he spent all his personal money on cigarettes, he would have to do without other things he might want, like new video games. That was a natural consequence. But if he put his hands on anyone in a physically aggressive manner, I would call the police. If he threatened, cursed, or intimidated caregivers, or if he made false accusations against staff, or destroyed property, he would be placed in a behavioral respite for a minimum of two weeks until he settled down and acted appropriately.

A behavior respite is simply a small facility where clients are closely supervised during their stay. There is no therapy involved; but rights are limited: no eating out or shopping, limited TV time, limited phone calls, locked doors; basically, clients are bored to death. If they misbehave while there, they incur a longer stay. This would be a consequence that I would impose because of aggressive behavior.

While no one liked to go to behavioral respite, John really hated it. He had ADHD and there was little to do and no place to go. He had to spend his time with others who threatened, destroyed property, and acted out. If no one else was there during his stay, he interacted only with staff. I told him it was his "thinking" time to get back on track. He knew why he had to go there. As he told me on several occasions, "God don't like ugly."

A big behavioral trigger for John is cell phones. Right now, I have three in my desk that I have confiscated from him. Two were purchased by him over the last few years, and one he stole when he ran away. When we found him and brought him home, he had a brand-new cell phone that he claimed an old girlfriend had given him. I knew it was untrue. And he knew I knew it was untrue. The problem is that I have no idea where he stole it, and he's not saying. John has personal spending money available to him each month, but it is limited, and he is a smoker, so most of his money goes for cigarettes after he purchases needed items. So given the opportunity, he may just take what he wants. He is clever enough not to suffer social consequences like everyone else, so except for what deterrents a conservator can impose, John has no reason to stop shop lifting.

I remember a situation when he was living with a provider family. They went to a restaurant for dinner and afterward, John ran off. Staff tried to follow, but he was evasive, ending up inside a nearby Walmart. He slipped some batteries into his pocket, then headed to sporting goods where he was confronted by the store's security guard. Knowing he was in serious trouble, John looked around, picked up a knife, and threatened to hurt himself. The guard backed away and called the police. The police spoke with John and his staff, who had arrived by that time, and then called me.

I told them what I knew. John was NOT going to hurt himself, that it was a ruse to get him into a psych hospital so he didn't have to go to jail. But the police must follow their protocols, so if someone threatens to hurt themselves, they must be taken to an emergency room. The ER has a protocol that says if someone threatens to hurt himself, they call in Mobile Crisis, who make a cursory evaluation and then—you guessed it—their protocol says they have the person referred to a psych hospital for further evaluation. If it is a good psych ward, they will usually release John within a few days, because they can recognize someone who is truly at risk and someone who has learned to play the system. In this situation, John went back home having had a three-day break and becoming energized from all the drama he caused. He chalked it up as a win. He got to eat lots of snacks, roam the halls, and chat up the new staff.

Back to cell phones. The issue is that John will call people repeatedly. A former foster mom told me he called her twenty-six times one day. This was his modus operandi; call repeatedly and leave multiple urgent messages. Then when someone finally gave in and picked up out of frustration, he told them he needed more money for cigarettes. Or a new video game. Or whatever.

One number he called often was the police. Never an emergency, but minor conflicts he had with his staff.

And he called me.

"Ron won't take me to play basketball," he said.

"Have you cleaned your room?"

"No."

"Clean your room and then he will take you."

"But I need to go play basketball now."

"Chores first, then basketball."

He hung up the phone.

Although he lost the first skirmish, John didn't give up. He rarely does.

Instead, he called the police. His story varied, but he usually told them that staff refused to feed him or had assaulted him. Metro police knew him. They spent countless hours dealing with "John" issues because of his easy access to them through his cell phone. Once he called them over something terrible staff had allegedly done to him, and by the time the officers arrived, he had gone to bed and was asleep. The drama was over.

Last week John got upset. He ran away, and when police picked him up claimed his staff had "beat him up." The police took him to the emergency room. The ER nurse called me.

"We have no reason to keep him," she told me. "But he says he won't go home."

John realized that they were going to send him home; but he wasn't ready to go. He told staff he had been beat up by his caregiver and that was why he couldn't go home. So, following protocol, they called adult protective services and the state investigative division for the mentally challenged. John told the investigator that he had marks on his body from the beating. (That was easily disproved; the bruises he claimed were nonexistent.)

But the first domino had fallen, and now John had to be removed from his home while a full-fledged investigation occurred. Staff couldn't work until the investigation was complete, which took about thirty days. There was no income for staff during that time, but there were tedious interviews, written statements, and other time consuming, stressful procedures just to prove that John, who had a well-documented history of making false allegations against caregivers, was lying and up to his old tricks.

After speaking with the investigator, I was furious. John, as usual, had spun a tall tale. And he would need a place to stay for a month while his caregiver was cleared. No way. I would not place him with someone else for his wanted "vacation." I called John.

"I am angry," I said. "I am tired of you making false allegations against people who are only trying to help you. This is what I want you to do. I will give you the investigator's name and phone number, and you will call and tell him the truth, do you understand? I don't want to hear excuses or explanations. False allegations and stirring up drama using hospitals and the police is the reason I took your phone away. If you *ever* want it back, you will call the investigator *now* on the house phone and tell the truth!"

No sound. Then I heard a soft, "Yes, ma'am. What is his number?"

I gave it to him, and to John's credit, he called immediately. The next thing I knew the investigation had been dropped. We were through until the next time. And there would be a next time.

Because of this long-standing pattern, one of the first actions I took as John's conservator concerned his cell phones. I told him I would take them away if certain conditions were not met. He had two pay-as-you-go phones at the time. He hollered, cursed, and carried on, but we made a written contract that included specific steps indicating responsible use had to be shown in order for him to keep them. He did not even fulfill the first step. I took the cell phones and put them in my desk. He simply didn't have the impulse control necessary to have unlimited access to a phone. He had access to a land line in his home but preferred not to use it because others could hear the tall tales he was telling.

When John made up a story accusing staff of mistreating him, he incurred no consequences. But he set wheels in motion, and a lot of time, money, and other resources were spent unnecessarily. So unless something dramatic happens, John will have no cell phone. And when he calls again to ask for his phones back, and I explain for the umpteenth time why that is not an option, he will get mad and hang up on me. On his landline.

Having a relationship with someone like John is a bit like a roller coaster ride. There are periods of relative calm, but they are brief, and the little boy sweetness is unexpected. On a good day, John sees me not as his guardian but as the one who always shows up when he is in trouble. A surrogate mother. The one who never goes away, even when he is at his worst. And he feels safe, I think, and protected. Not just from the outside world but from himself.

At these times, he wants to show appreciation, much like a child will pick a dandelion for his mom. I have received various gifts from John through the years. Nothing expensive. A mug with his photo on it, probably given to him. A used speaker that no longer worked. Half a package of candy. Recently he gave me a small bottle of blue hand sanitizer. Nothing he would buy, but something he might steal. Should I confront him, demand to know where he got it? Give him another lecture on shop lifting? Make him take it back?

But I saw his face. So eager for approval, and love. He watched me, waiting to see how I would respond.

"How nice of you to think of me," I said. "What a sweet gift."

His face broke into a smile, and he grabbed me in a bear hug.

"I love you, Miss Belinda."

"I love you too," I told him as he walked away, smiling.

I sighed.

John's impulsiveness resulted in lots of poor decisions. One of his many caregivers was a petite, middle-aged female caregiver. She called me one night.

"Miss Belinda." The voice sounded urgent.

"Yes? What's going on?"

"John is angry, and he's ripping up all his clothes."

"Where are you?"

"I locked myself in my room."

"OK. I have never known John to hurt a woman, so I don't think you're in any danger. But just stay in there. Where is he right now?"

"In the kitchen. He dumped all his clothes on the floor and starting yelling and tearing them up."

"Has John destroyed anything of yours?"

"No, just his own clothes."

"Do you know what started this?"

"He said his girlfriend broke up with him, and he wanted to tear up the shirt she gave him. What should I do?"

"Stay in your room for now. Don't confront him. Leave him alone. Let him tear up everything he owns."

"Should I call the police?"

"Not unless he starts destroying *your* property. Try to let it play out."

As I spoke, I processed this in my head. The caregiver was a small woman, and John used that to his advantage. He would physically threaten her, and at his size he had a huge advantage. He was on a rampage in her small apartment, and she was feeling helpless. John could easily break down her door if he chose, but I didn't think he would. He operated by a self-imposed rule that said a man can't hit a woman. Threaten, yes, but he can't touch her. But then I remembered once when he got mad, he tore a bedroom door off its hinges and slung it down a hallway, leaving huge scratch marks on the wooden floor. That was right after he picked up his television and threw it across the room. And a few times he had assaulted a roommate.

I stayed on the phone with her, realizing that just staying connected gave us both some reassurance.

Eventually, John settled down and, leaving the pile of clothes in the middle of the kitchen floor, went to bed.

Early the next morning I got a call.

"Miss Belinda."

"Hi, John."

"Can I ask you something?"

I braced myself. This is how most of his calls started.

"Sure."

"Can you buy me some new clothes?"

"New clothes? Why do you need new clothes?"

"Now don't get mad. My clothes got tore up last night."

"What do you mean, torn up?"

"They're all ripped up."

"Ripped up?"

"Well, here's what happened. My girlfriend broke up with me."

"Okaaayyy."

"Miss Belinda, I'll be honest with you. I got mad and tore up the shirt she gave me."

"I get it. But what about your other clothes?"

"I tore them up, too. Please, can we go shopping? I don't have anything to wear."

"Hmmm. You have a problem, John."

"What do you mean?"

"You just told me you got angry and deliberately tore up all of your clothes. Is that right?"

"Yes, but Miss Belinda, I was mad. I couldn't help it."

"Well, remember we talked about our choices having consequences?"

He saw where this conversation was headed.

"But I don't have anything to wear!"

"Wow, John. What are you going to do?"

"I. Need. To. Go. Shopping."

"I don't think so, John."

"BUT I HAVE NOTHING TO WEAR!"

"It seems to me you have two choices: you can either select something you have ripped or you can go naked. Call me tomorrow and let me know what you decided. Bye!"

As I hung up the phone, I was hoping he wouldn't walk out in his birthday suit just to "show me." It would totally freak out his caregiver and prompt the neighbors to call the police.

But he found something to wear that day, and over the next few weeks we replaced a few shirts and pairs of shorts—from Goodwill. And he remembered that incident and assured me over and over it would never happen again.

"I learnt my lesson good, Miss Belinda. Next time I'll just tear up the shirt she gave me and leave the other clothes alone."

"Good decision, John. That is a much more mature response."

He smiled sheepishly.

I knew that although John was calm in the courtroom when the conservatorship was granted, it wouldn't be long until he tested me. I expected him to blow up, maybe break a few items, threaten his staff. I was prepared to have him placed in a behavioral respite when that occurred. He needed immediate consequences to assist him in controlling his behavior. For too long he had used his size and threats to control his staff. He had the mind of a child and needed to feel secure, to know that someone was in charge.

I didn't have to wait long. Only a few weeks later he was intimidating staff, refusing to bathe or take his medications as prescribed, and fighting with his roommate. The director of his provider agency and I called him to the office to talk about what was going on. As I expected, he was defiant, blaming everyone else for his actions. Then he demanded his cell phone back.

"John, I don't have it with me. But even if I did, do you remember why I took it away?"

"You said I called people too many times."

"Yes, and we also talked about how often you call police, making false accusations against staff. Remember our contract? You can get it back when you decide to follow the contract."

John glared at me. He was getting worked up. He knew the director and I wanted to talk about his recent aggressive behavior, and he was trying to deflect. (Later, I found out he had bought a prepaid cell phone by pawning some of his video game equipment. It was in his pocket at the time.)

He became more and more belligerent.

"It's MY phone, so give it back!" he shouted.

"That's not why we're here. What's going on at home?"

"Nothing." He slumped down in his chair and crossed his arms. He stared at me.

"Come on, John. We want to hear your side of things."

"I don't have to talk to you. I want my phone back."

I looked over at the director who spoke up, calmly urging him to talk to us. He refused, keeping his arms crossed and staring straight ahead. I spoke again.

"OK John, you don't have to say anything. But please listen carefully."

He continued to stare straight ahead with his arms folded, slouched down in the chair.

"Your behavior, over the last month or so has been totally unacceptable. You are threatening your staff, refusing to cooperate, and making life miserable for everyone around you, including your roommate. You are constantly trying to pick a fight. It must stop. I am sending you to behavior respite for a few weeks to help you get control again and change your behavior."

I barely gotten the words out of my mouth before he sat up straight in his chair and exploded.

"I AM NOT GOING TO BEHAVIOR RESPITE," he yelled. "I WILL GO TO JAIL FIRST!"

With that, John suddenly jumped up, ran down the hall and out the front door. I followed him. His eyes fell on his caregiver's car parked nearby. He ran over, kicked a big dent in the passenger side door, and then put his fist through the window. Glass scattered everywhere.

Shaking blood off his right hand, he turned around and headed back toward the office. He kicked in the glass front door, stepped through into the hall, and checked out the first doorway. It was the conference room. He twisted a 48-inch wall TV from its metal frame, threw it on the floor, then stomped on it with his size 12 shoes. Seeing nothing else in the room except a table and chairs, he continued down the hallway. At the end of the hallway was the common workspace for the agency. His eyes lit up.

John grabbed the printer and threw it on the floor, stomping it after it hit the ground. Then he saw the fax machine, and it went down too. Computer screen, keyboard—everything electronic hit the floor and got stomped on. I stood in the doorway watching, but not trying to stop him. I didn't want anyone hurt, and I knew this had to play out. Telephone, answering machine, Keurig, water cooler. Then he saw his caregiver, whose car he had just damaged, peering around a corner. He ran over and yanked her cell phone out of her hands and threw it on the floor. He left small blood smears on different objects around the room as he continued to pick up and toss whatever he saw.

I didn't see the director, but I was sure she was on a call to the police. The others in the office had quickly exited and were waiting outside until they arrived.

I followed John through the suite of offices but stayed about six to eight feet away. Standing in the doorways, I watched as he destroyed more and more property. So, this was my test. This was where he let me know in no uncertain terms that he was *not* happy about having a conservator; he would make his *own* decisions and do as he pleased. He was not using his voice but his hands, and his feet, and his entire body to let me know he was still in charge. And to see if he could scare me.

John was a really big guy, but I was not afraid of him. I knew he could hurt me, badly, if he chose. But I believed I had established enough of a relationship with him through the years that he would not *deliberately* hurt me. He felt protective of me and had even offered to be my bodyguard if I ever needed him. He once demonstrated how he would break someone's shins if they tried to harm me. That was part of the deal we had made a few years earlier to stop his physical violence. He promised to never assault anyone again if I promised to call him if I ever needed a bodyguard. We shook hands on it.

Besides, in a calm moment right after I became his conservator, we were discussing his aggressive behavior, and I told him in no uncertain terms that if he ever "laid his hands on me" I would press charges and have him put in jail. That was the line I drew in the sand.

By now this property destruction rampage had been going on about ten minutes, and the agency offices were a mess. The building tenants from down the hall had heard what was going on and were frightened. There was a barber shop, beauty shop, and other small businesses on our floor. A few of the owners had stepped into the hall with makeshift weapons, whatever they could pick up to protect themselves. Two of the men kept trying to get me to hide in their offices. They were concerned that I was a woman and John was out of control. I had trouble convincing them that I was safer than they were.

Thinking that maybe the incident had about run its course and John's impulsive anger was cooling down, I went back into the office hallway. I stepped out in front of him as he exited the conference room, looking for something else to destroy.

"John," I said calmly. "Don't you think you've done enough?"

Before I could continue, he shoved me against the wall, towering over me by almost nine inches. I looked up into his face and saw his startled expression. It couldn't have been plainer had he spoken the words out loud. Oh, no. I put my hands on Miss Belinda.

Backing away, he quickly retraced his steps. So he wasn't through yet. I leaned against the door jamb, watching his face as he scoured the next room. He had already destroyed or damaged most everything in it. Then his expression brightened. Striding across the room, he grabbed the fire extinguisher off the wall.

His caregiver came around the corner, and she got sprayed first. I turned and started quickly walking away. He followed me a few steps, spraying my back, then hesitated and glanced into a nearby office. He slowly sprayed every surface in the room, then walked to the next office. He did the same to every room he entered until the extinguisher was empty. Every surface was covered with a fine, powdery mess.

At last, John went into a back office and locked the door. I walked outside to see if the police had arrived just as two patrol cars and an EMT unit rolled up. His caregiver was treated for inhalation due to being sprayed in the face by the fire extinguisher. But no one else was hurt.

The police retrieved John from the locked office and placed him in the back of the patrol car. Although he was calm now, he was still defiant. I walked over to the car.

"I told you I'm not going to behavior respite," he smirked.

"Yes, yes, you are. As soon as you get out of jail," I replied matter-of-factly.

The next day, John called me from the county jail.

"Miss Belinda."

"Yes?"

"What time are you going to bail me out today?"

"I'm not."

"What do you mean?"

"I'm not going to bail you out."

"But you have to. Someone always bails me out."

"Maybe that's part of the problem."

"But I can't stay in here."

"It's only for a few days, John, until your preliminary hearing."

"Puleeease, Miss Belinda. It's only a few hundred dollars."

"Do you have any money, John?"

"No. You can use yours."

"You destroyed an entire office because you were mad and have been charged with a felony. You shoved me against a wall, which is a misdemeanor. Now you want me to spend my money to get you out of jail early? I don't think so."

He hung up the phone. But the next day he called again.

"Miss Belinda,"

"Yes, John."

"Can you call the sheriff's office and ask them to get me an extra blanket? It's cold in here."

"No, John, I won't call the sheriff's office to get you an extra blanket."

"But what if I get sick?"

"You won't get sick. It's not that cold."

"But I can't sleep."

"Well, that's okay. You can lie there and think about what put you in jail."

He hung up the phone again.

He ended up staying a total of ten days in a county jail. Even though John was intellectually challenged, he was not only huge but street smart. I didn't see him as vulnerable in the county jail. As I expected, nobody messed with him because of his size and the fact that everyone knew something was a little off. When we got to court, the judge put him on probation and let him go on the condition he went straight to behavioral respite, like we had originally planned. He was not happy but had no choice. He was sent several counties over to a new respite, one with which I was unfamiliar. The one John dreaded so much had no empty beds.

At respite he lasted three days before they took him to an emergency room . . . for bad behavior. They said he was being physically aggressive, and they wanted him transferred to a psych hospital. But there was no psychosis, no mental breakdown. The behavioral respite didn't want to deal with him, even though that was their job. And the psych hospital that the ER transferred him too soon figured this out. John didn't belong there. He teased with the staff. Ate lots of snacks. Watched a lot of TV. According to John, "This place ain't that bad."

I am familiar with three behavioral respite facilities. Each one cares for only a handful of clients at a time. The goal is not to rehabilitate but to provide a "timeout" for the client and hope they calm down and can return to their normal living pattern.

Unfortunately, the same clients seem to cycle through again and again because no changes are being made. The staff are poorly paid for the work they do and take physical risks every time they walk in the door.

Not until the Rehabilitation Act of 1973 were the rights of people with disabilities protected by law. Since that time, other laws have been passed to expand those rights. Among those who receive services for their intellectual disabilities, personal rights have been emphasized so they can not only advocate for themselves but have a better quality of life. The passing of the Rehabilitation Act was way overdue; other groups had been recognized years earlier with Title VI of the Civil Rights Act.

But one unintended consequence of clients being reminded repeatedly of their rights was that many, like John, didn't understand that along with rights there were responsibilities. John thought only of his own rights and would run roughshod over the rights of others. Many of those supported by the state who had moderate to mild intellectual disabilities did the same thing, being physically or verbally aggressive.

Staff were so well trained on their client's rights that they often allowed themselves to be mistreated. I regularly reminded both staff and clients of the basic principle that "my rights stop where your rights start." Those with disabilities do not have the right to mistreat the people who are caring for them. The purpose of legislation has been to "equalize" opportunities and quality of life for those who are at a disadvantage. It was not intended to do so at the expense of others. We should lift each other up and support each other commensurate with our abilities and resources.

CHAPTER 5

Taking Risks

Social work is not for the faint-hearted. Anyone who has been a social worker for any length of time has been in uncomfortable, potentially dangerous, or outright dangerous situations. And especially if you do mental health crisis work, you are always aware of the possibility that someone may get out of control and hurt you, either deliberately or accidentally. Every mental health worker must personally decide how to handle the risk.

I choose faith. Not a "nothing can happen to me" kind of faith, but rather the faith that says God has this. Whatever happens, God has this.

My twenty-something-year-old son doesn't fully agree with my philosophy. He thinks I need a way to protect myself. I respect and appreciate where he is coming from. At seventeen, he was the victim of a violent, FBI-investigated hate crime. He was abducted on a rural road at night by two men he didn't know, beaten up, and left unconscious in an open field. It happened two days before Christmas and was terrifying. The experience left him with a concussion, years of memory issues, and post-traumatic stress disorder.

. He approached me one day and suggested I get a license to carry a gun.

"No," I said. "No gun. I have always been nonviolent, and I don't intend to ever carry a gun."

"A knife, then."

"No, son, I won't carry a knife." I smiled. "Well, come to think of it, I have a pocketknife in my purse. Your granddaddy gave it to me a long time ago."

"Mom. That won't do much. But the law says that four-inch knives are now legal."

"How do you even know that?"

"I just know. Come on, Mom, you have to be able to protect yourself. At least buy some mace."

"No. Andrew. Listen, I am not stupid. I know something bad can happen. But every time I look at that mace I will be reminded of my fear. And if I focus on that I can't do my job."

He looked at me with a mixture of disgust and incredulity, then walked away. I thought the attempt to persuade me to carry a weapon was over. I was wrong.

A few days later, I walked to my car and headed to work. When I opened the door, I saw a pair of nunchucks lying on the driver's seat. I knew they were Andrew's. He had collected swords and other Ninja weapons since he was a young teen. I picked them up and walked back inside the house.

"Look what I found," I said.

"I know," he replied. "They're nunchucks."

"But why are they in my car?"

"Because you won't use a knife or gun and you need something to protect yourself."

I laughed out loud. Japanese nunchucks can be described as a weapon consisting of two, foot-long wooden or metal sticks joined by a chain. The idea is to protect yourself against assault by holding one long stick in your hand and swinging the chain through the air and over your head. You make contact against your assailant with the other stick, knocking him out cold.

Andrew did not appreciate my laughter.

I tried to explain. "There's a problem," I said. "If I swing that thing in a circle over my head, there is a good chance I will knock *myself* out!"

He looked at me, shook his head, and just walked away.

I loved him for caring and wanting to protect me. And I must admit I felt pretty good that he thought his gray-haired mother of five could effectively use a Japanese attack weapon.

Although I choose not to carry a weapon of any kind, I try to use sound judgment by exercising caution and thinking ahead. There are neighborhoods I stay out of after dark, and I try to always be aware of my surroundings. There have been times that I felt uncomfortable before I even got out of the car, and I just drove away to come back another day. I have learned to listen to my instincts, and clients themselves have warned me to leave their homes and neighborhoods before dark. On a few occasions, I have called for police backup, although I remember sometimes the officers were more afraid than I was.

A young coworker and I needed to extract an intellectually challenged man with cerebral palsy from a home where his caregivers were two family members—a heroin addict and a registered sex offender. There was also a chance the addict's supplier was with them. We had the necessary court papers, but knowing it might get a little dicey, I called for police backup before we arrived at the house. When I gave the office the address, he sounded uneasy.

"I know that house," he said. "And I'm getting ready to retire soon. I'd like to be able to make it till then. Let me call for back up."

We waited outside the front gate of the house until first one patrol car and then another arrived. The officers conferred while my coworker and I stood nearby. They made no move to acknowledge us. After a few minutes I approached them to explain the situation.

"The man we are bringing out will be in a wheelchair," I told them. "He lives in squalor and has no belongings worth saving so we should be in and out pretty quickly. But some of his family are upset so we thought it better to have y'all here."

The older officer nodded; the younger one looked toward the house. We stood there awkwardly, the four of us. After some silence it became obvious the officers were in no hurry to enter. They were waiting on us to act first. I turned to my coworker.

"Lorie, are you ready? Let's go bring Max out."

I looked toward the officers. They waited without moving or speaking.

"See that front door?" I asked the officers, pointing toward the house. "When we go in I will leave that door open. Please keep your eyes on it. If we need help, I will come to the door and wave to you to come in. OK?"

"Okay," said the older officer. He looked relieved. I'm sure he was hoping he wasn't needed. So was I.

The younger one shifted uncomfortably where he stood and stared down the street, away from the house. He didn't say a word, and he never looked me in the face.

We were able to remove Max from the house and load him and his wheelchair into the car without needing their assistance. One of his caregivers was angry and confrontational but made no physical move to stop us. The other was lying on the sofa in a drug stupor. She mumbled something about being glad we were taking him to a better place. A quick thought raced through my head. I wish we could take *her* to a better place. She needed help, too.

I learned something valuable that day. Everyone is afraid, even seasoned police officers who are trained to handle volatile situations. Those in professions which put them at risk just simply try to move through it. And there is another important principle I learned early in my career: never show your fear. It gives an unstable opponent an advantage.

As I sit here typing, I am painfully aware of my swollen black eye. It happened when I was trying to restrain a skinny, six-foot tall man from hurting himself. Another battle scar. They don't tell you about this in college.

A memory pops up: the time a mentally ill man became paranoid and thought I was trying to hurt him. In his mind I was conspiring with his father who lived in another state. It had something to do with money, but I never understood exactly what he was angry about. He just thought I was out to get him. He wouldn't accept the fact that I didn't know his father and had never had any kind of contact with him. I was working in my office on unending paperwork when our secretary came to the door. She looked worried.

"There's a man walking up and down the halls looking for you," she said. "And he's upset. I didn't tell him where you were."

"What does he look like?" I asked.

"Average height, in his twenties, olive skin. I think something is off."

"Oh. I think I know who that is."

When I first started trying to help Anthony, red flags went off and I googled him. One of the things that came up in my search was an out-of-state mugshot for assault. The Internet has its advantages.

I met him and his mom on a quick run to the grocery store on a Christmas Eve. They were living out of their car. I invited them to our home for dinner, and they came. They used my washer and dryer to do their laundry, and I offered them a bedroom to sleep in that night. The mother just smiled and told me they were going to midnight Christmas mass. They never returned, but I had given them my business card and referred them to someone who could help with her medical bills. Much later I found out they had gotten over $1000 for medical expenses from my referral. That was months ago. So why was he looking for me now?

"Maggie," I asked the secretary, "how did he get in?"

She said he had followed behind an employee as she entered the building with her punch code.

After stopping at the secretary's office, Anthony started down the hall, looking through the glass window in every office, searching for me. He was angry and muttering to himself. My boss made me hide behind a door in her office until he gave up and left. I was asked to stay home for a few days until he settled down. No need to scare my coworkers. He came back a second time and the police were called, but he left before they arrived. Thankfully, I wasn't there.

That was the last I heard of him. Perhaps medication mitigated his psychosis. I hope so.

CBS News reported in 2017 that The Bureau of Labor Statistics listed the twenty deadliest civilian jobs in the United States (cbsnews.com/pictures/the-20-deadliest-jobs-in-America-ranked/). Social work came in at number twenty. As a basis of comparison, firefighters and police officers ranked fifteenth, with logging being listed as number one. According to the Occupational Health and Safety Administration, 70 to 74 percent of all workplace assaults occurred in the fields of healthcare and social services. The Bureau of Labor Statistics reported that healthcare and social service workers were four times more likely than the general population to become a victim of those assaults.

In addition to the physical risks involved, there is often a mental price to pay. Burnout is common, and stress related illnesses take their toll: anxiety disorders, depression, even PTSD. Compassion fatigue is a common characteristic of burn out. Interacting with people face to face in their life crises is draining emotionally, and you can't leave it at work; you carry it home with you. You go to sleep with it on your mind, and you wake up with it still there. Sometimes you dream about it.

Each client and each situation is different from the last and brings a new set of challenges. There is no rule book to follow, no step-by-step manual, no lesson plan. There is never a *single* problem to address but rather *multiple* issues radiating out from the problem you were called to deal with. Nothing is simple, nothing can be addressed with finality when dealing with mental health. It's a lot like playing whack-a-mole at an arcade. You knock down one problem and another immediately springs up. With much experience, practice, and determination (and a reasonable caseload) you can almost keep up. Almost. But the game never ends.

CHAPTER 6

The Girl Who Swallowed Office Supplies

Jessica had an unusual habit. She swallowed office supplies. Things like push pins and paper clips. Pen caps and thumb tacks. But that's not all she swallowed.

Jessica would swallow just about anything that would fit down her throat. In the three years I worked with her, she made dozens of trips to emergency rooms because of swallowed objects. Staff had to watch her constantly; she would break a cup or glass and swallow small pieces. She would disassemble a pen and swallow the cap, or the spring. She would take caps off condiments from the refrigerator and gulp them down. Nothing was hung on her wall, because she would swallow the nail or picture hanger that held it there. Her eyes were constantly searching for things to swallow. Keys, small pieces of jewelry, bobby pens; nothing was off limits. Once shc swallowed the plastic bolt cover from a toilet seat. She swallowed hair clips, bottle caps. When nothing else was available to swallow, she would rip small pieces from her heavy plastic shower curtain and down her throat they'd go.

Outdoors it was just as bad. She would pick up small pieces of glass, soda can tabs, even small rocks if that was all she could find. She was assigned two staff to work with her since someone had to have eyes on her every minute. They were with her every time she left her house, one on each side, to keep her safe from her potentially deadly habit. Each staff looped her arm through Jessica's, but she learned to scour the ground furtively while talking and laughing. Then suddenly, she would yank an arm free and lean over and grab whatever it was she had seen. Her quickness usually caught them off guard and it would be in her mouth before staff even had time to respond. Then the challenge was to get the item out of her mouth before she swallowed it. Rarely were they successful, and most of the time it meant another trip to the ER.

But that too often failed. While she was waiting to be seen, Jessica would look for something else to swallow. One time, I watched as she quickly approached the nurses' station and lunged over the counter to pick up some small stationary item no one had noticed but her. Down her throat it went.

The amazing thing was that the hospital rarely had to do anything but X-ray her and tell staff to watch for it to leave her body via her poop. She swallowed things easily, and her esophagus was never perforated, nothing ever got stuck. Things were passed from her stomach to her colon and

traveled through her body until they exited on their own. Staff had to don gloves and be on the lookout.

One day, I received a report that Jessica had swallowed a screw. She was taken to the ER and was X-rayed to make sure no damage had been done. They e-mailed me a copy. I was shocked. There, plain as day, was a three-inch-long screw. But she was, once again, unharmed. The doctor simply threaded a magnetic scope down her throat and pulled it out.

No one really knew what caused this behavior. Jessica didn't have Pica (a condition that compels one to eat inedible objects.) She was diagnosed with borderline personality disorder and an intellectual disability. In my opinion, I believe her swallowing may have started as a way not only to get attention but also for the sheer drama it caused. That desire for drama is often characteristic of her disorder. Over time, Jessica's habit took on a life of its own. With an average emergency room bill of $1500 plus, dozens of ER visits cost the taxpayers plenty. Doctors bill separately, and ambulances were sometimes involved, so the actual cost was much higher. The day would come when Jessica would swallow something that might put her life in danger or kill her. Something needed to be done to keep her safe.

I tried to get a conservator appointed for her. Without one, Jessica could, and did, refuse treatment that her support team recommended. She refused to cooperate, with no repercussions or consequences at all. She *liked* swallowing things. It brought her lots of attention.

Our team member representative from the state, who knew her well, agreed she needed one. Her staff agreed. Her provider agency agreed. I talked to a professional friend familiar with her issues, and she agreed to be her pro bono conservator. Jessica knew and liked her, and *she* agreed. I was elated. We were finally moving forward after years of trying to find a good solution to the problem. We scheduled a meeting to discuss the conservatorship and proceed. I prepared data to make the case for Jessica to have a conservator just in case there was someone present at the meeting who was against the idea. As it turned out, there were two people present who were against the plan. One was a state psychologist; the other was a paid advocate. They were concerned that her rights were being taken away.

I pulled out my data sheet and read aloud some of the statistics, focusing on the number of items swallowed and the emergency room trips that followed. I even detailed some of the scariest items she had swallowed. The advocate spoke first. He was against it, he said, because conservatorship would restrict her rights.

"Yes," I said, "but she is not safe. And health and safety have to be our priority here. One day she may swallow something that kills her."

He shook his head. "I am not in favor of this," he repeated. "I don't think we should take away any of her rights."

The state psychologist had been sitting quietly. Now he spoke. "I agree," he said. "I see no need to take her rights away."

"But the data," I said. "Hundreds of these incidents required ER trips. I can't believe she has not been severely hurt already. We have to act now to protect her from herself. That's our job."

"She's not at risk."

"What??" I couldn't believe my ears. "She's not at risk? I just presented the facts. How can you say that?"

"She's not at risk," he repeated.

This was pure nonsense. He might as well have said the moon is not round. Data, witnesses, reports, facts. All were present. This representative of the state agency, to whom taxpayers had entrusted Jessica's safety, chose to ignore the data. Her minimum wage daily caregiver would have made a better decision.

Once the state psychologist spoke, the discussion, for all practical purposes, was over. No one wanted to contradict him. No one wanted to rock the boat, so there would be no conservatorship. Jessica would continue to swallow anything she could get her hands on. She would not be required to participate in any type of therapy or program that might help. The decision would be left to her. And we knew what she would do—refuse and continue to swallow.

It was, and still is, as far as I know, a lawsuit waiting to happen. I documented everything in case something awful ever happened to Jessica on my watch and the state tried to blame me for neglect.

Jessica had other issues, too. At times she was violent; it usually was a caregiver or a police officer on the receiving end of her aggression. She spat on, kicked, and struck anyone who was trying to manage her behavior. Once she was under control, she found other ways to voice her displeasure. She would urinate on herself deliberately and pull scabs off her arms and legs to make them bleed.

Jessica has spent her life crying out for help.

CHAPTER 7

Conservatorship

Conservatorship is a sticky issue among those who advocate for people with intellectual and mental health disabilities. The person deemed incompetent to manage his own affairs may have his rights taken away and given to someone who has been judged capable by the court to manage them responsibly. From time to time, we see something in the news about conservatorship, usually when one has gone wrong or is being contested. Britney Spears' conservator issues have been in the news off and on for years.

Conservatorship isn't a one-size-fits-all legal agreement. Depending on the situation, a judge may grant legal power over a person's finances or medical care only; or the conservator may be granted full power over an individual, which would include managing all living arrangements and necessities such as food, clothing and shelter, legal affairs, and supervision.

Sometimes this is done with the person's approval, sometimes without.

In my personal experience, courts take this responsibility very seriously, and while I am sure there are conservators who do not always follow their client's best interests, for most in my field, anyway, it is a thankless job. Conservators are doing both their clients and society at large a service. But many Internet bloggers and organized groups are quite vocal in their opposition to any type of conservatorship. I learned that firsthand about eleven years ago when I became conservator in a local, high visibility situation.

Rights are only intended to be restricted when the person cannot, due to lack of ability or impeded by a mental illness, perform normal activities involved in daily living on their own. A court hearing is required with all parties present, and the petition for conservatorship may be either granted or denied, but only after all points of view have been heard and evidence considered. Sometimes, especially with children, the court will appoint an independent guardian ad litem. This appointment is only for the legal action presently occurring and is usually an attorney. The guardian's job is to check into the facts of the case, working toward the best interest of the child or adult facing guardianship. Then they make a report to the judge while conservatorship is being considered. By its very nature, appointing a conservator is subjective, even though based on evidence and testimony. The court will not appoint a conservator just because a person makes bad decisions. All of us fall into that category from time to time.

But a mental illness or lack of mental capacity puts the affected person into a different category. They not only make bad decisions from time to time, they *live* there. And their bad decisions make them unable to care for their own health or safety. To complicate things further, their mental state and/or disability make(s) them more vulnerable. They are unable to resist fraud or undue influence. Part of a conservator's responsibility is to protect them from being taken advantage of.

When a child with a disability turns eighteen, most state laws say he is officially a legal adult, regardless of his ability to independently handle his own affairs. At this point, a parent loses the right to see medical records, determine medical care, make educational or treatment decisions, or make living arrangements. Even if the mentally disabled child has an IQ of 37, the parents no longer are legally allowed to make decisions for that child. As a result, parents must spend a lot of time and money hiring an attorney to petition the court for guardianship over their own child. In my opinion, whether living at home with family or supported by the state, every person who is not capable of living independently due to cognitive or mental health issues should have a legal conservator. It both prevents and solves a lot of problems that will certainly come up.

Charles was a great example of this. I was his case worker, and he had no conservator. I tried to deal with his health insurance provider over the phone. She would give me no information because I was not his conservator. I introduced myself and the conversation began.

"How can I help you?"

"I need to talk to you about Charles' health coverage. He is having some issues with his insurance. I am his caseworker."

"I will need to talk to him directly."

"Ma'am, that is not possible. Charles is profoundly intellectually challenged and cannot understand what you are saying. He speaks only a few words, and they are not intelligible."

"Is he over eighteen?"

"Yes, he is forty-one."

"Then he will have to sign a release saying I can talk to you about his health insurance."

"No ma'am, he can't do that. He has severe cerebral palsy and cannot even hold a pencil."

"Well, let him make his X and you can write his name in beside the X. I will send you the release."

"I just explained that he cannot hold a pencil. He does not know what an 'X' is and has no concept of letters or what they represent."

This went on a few more minutes, each of us repeating what we had already said. I became more frustrated as the conversation went on.

She would not give in and could offer no other way for me *as his caseworker* to resolve the issue. So, I went to his house with the form she mailed me. I forced his stiff fingers around the pen, and I made a scraggly "X." Charles thought it was a game and laughed as I struggled to control his spastic hand.

The next time I called, the insurance representative was delighted. She had her "signature" on file, and we were able to resolve his insurance problem.

When someone who is intellectually challenged is enrolled in a state program to receive full lifetime medical and financial care, like the State of Tennessee offers, the court should automatically be petitioned for a conservator. To me this is a no-brainer, since the main criteria for being admitted to the program is lack of ability to care for oneself independently due to lack of capacity. Both federal and state tax monies are used to pay for these wonderful services and taxpayers need to know resources are being used wisely.

The responsibility given to a conservator is great and should not be taken on lightly. The conservator is responsible to the court for all his actions on behalf of his client. In addition to the high degree of accountability, there is a lot of paperwork and filing required. A conservator has a legal agreement with the court to provide whatever services fall within the wording of the court order and in a timely manner. He also has an ethical and moral responsibility to put his client's interests above his own.

Conservators are usually paid out of the person's estate at a rate approved by the court. I personally choose not to accept any fees or file for out-of-pocket expenses for my wards. There are several reasons for this. First, most clients in my field don't have any money except social security benefits. Second, it is not a full-time job for me, but rather a volunteer service. And third, conservatorships can be controversial.

I have had a couple of situations where families lost conservatorship due to neglect or abuse, and I was appointed in their place. The first thing they accused me of was "doing it for the money." Since I cannot eliminate the adversarial relationship that I often have with families of my wards, I thought to minimize them by removing the money motive.

If all I did was manage clients through conservatorship, I would not have the option of refusing payment for services. It is an honorable profession. But since I choose to do this on a volunteer basis, I do my work pro bono. That eliminates lots of problems with families, and there is a bonus. When I volunteer my services, I find that sometimes others do, too. Attorneys donate many hours on behalf of my clients. On the downside, I cannot manage more than a few at a time and still fulfill my other responsibilities.

CHAPTER 8

I Am a Rat

Britney was sexually abused as child. She was eventually diagnosed with both an intellectual disability and schizophrenia and has had too many psychotic episodes to remember. On one occasion staff called me with an urgent request. Could I come over immediately?

When I arrived about twenty minutes later, Britney was standing in the middle of her small kitchen, staring at the floor. She had opened all the cabinets and emptied the contents. Cans of vegetables, boxes of mac and cheese, spices, and assorted food items were all over the kitchen tile.

"Hey Britney," I said. "Why is all this stuff on the floor?"

She didn't look at me.

"Britney?"

She spoke softly. "Because I'm a rat," she replied, eyes still downcast. "And rats eat off the floor."

"Oh Britney," I said, touching her arm lightly. "You are definitely not a rat. You are a beautiful young woman."

"No, I'm not." she said, pulling back from me, but keeping her eyes on the floor. "I am a rat."

Britney's self-image was only one of many problems she had to deal with. She was afraid of monsters hiding under her bed, and at times she would say she saw them. As I came to understand her hallucinations better, I knew she did see them, even though no one else could. We had a solid, wooden bed frame built to the floor and placed her mattress on top. Britney saw that nothing could fit under the bed, including monsters. This helped some. Up until then she would carry her comforter to the sofa and sleep out near her overnight awake staff. She didn't want to be alone.

Sometimes Britney became violent, both toward herself and others. With two staff assigned to her home, we could usually keep her roommate safe and out of the way, but we had to figure out ways to keep Britney safe during these episodes. To keep her from breaking mirrors, we installed plexiglass over them so they would not shatter when she threw things at them. For a time, we placed her television in a plexiglass box for the same reason. She erupted without much notice, so two staff were required in her home during waking hours. Even when she was not having a violent episode, eyes had to be on her all the time. She would sneak out the front door, strip, and sit on the curb in front of her house, all 250 pounds of her. Neighbors loved it when she did that.

Britney had been on a psych ward for two weeks. I went to see her, and a nurse met me at the door.

"I'm so glad you're here," she said. "We can't do anything with her. Can you calm her down?"

"What is she doing?"

"She is running up and down the halls naked. She won't put her clothes on."

"Is she hearing voices?" I asked.

"I didn't know she heard voices."

"She's schizophrenic," I replied. "Check her chart."

The head nurse walked up.

"Did you know Britney hears voices?" the first nurse asked her. The head nurse shook her head.

I couldn't believe what I was hearing. Two full weeks in a psych hospital and no one paid attention to her diagnosis? No one knew she hallucinated?

"Tell Britney that Miss Belinda is here. Tell her to put her clothes on and we will have a visit."

I went down the hall to a small visiting area and waited. In a few minutes Britney came shuffling down the hall toward me, unkempt, wild-eyed but wearing a loose-hanging dress. She wore no shoes, and it appeared she had on no undergarments either. The nurse was nervous. She propped the door open, then hurried out.

"Hey, Britney. Have a seat," I motioned to the sofa. She sat down and I pulled a chair up close to her. Britney always cared about how she looked, and right now she looked a mess. I sensed she was tightly wound and that I didn't have all her attention. She was in her own head.

"Britney," I said, thinking I might be able to help her refocus on the present, "Britney, I know you got dressed in a hurry. Here, I have a comb. Let's make you pretty. Maybe some lipstick?"

The face in front of me suddenly crumpled; her body seemed to shrink back into itself. A thin, whiny, little girl's voice spoke out of Britney's mouth. She looked at me defiantly.

"Why are you trying to make me wear makeup?" she asked. "I'm just a little girl."

I sat there, stunned. Britney was in her early thirties. I couldn't believe what I was hearing.

"I'm sorry, Britney. Of course you don't have to wear makeup if you don't want to. But you are an adult woman. You're not a little girl anymore."

She raised her voice. "I am *not* a grownup," she said, "I'm a little girl. Little girls don't wear lipstick."

I stopped talking and just observed her. For a few moments, we sat there in silence. Then she suddenly stiffened, and her body told me something was coming. Her face contorted.

"Don't talk to her like that," boomed a new, deeper voice. "Don't tell her she's not a little girl because she is." The voice was strong, almost fierce, and spoke with authority. It wasn't Britney's voice, nor did it belong to the little girl.

"Who are you?" I asked.

"You know me," she admonished, rather sternly. "You know me."

"I'm afraid I don't," I said, "so you must tell me. What is your name?"

Silence.

"Please, what is your name?"

Suddenly, she bellowed. "MY NAME IS BLOODY MARY! MY NAME IS BLOODY MARY!"

I sat there, astonished at what I was hearing. Britney's whole demeanor had changed. She was sitting on the edge of the sofa now, staring at me as if she didn't know with whom she was conversing. She looked belligerent, not at all like Britney, or even the little girl. She looked crazed and unfocused. I said nothing but watched her face. She sat perfectly still, as if she was frozen. I was the first to speak.

“I don’t understand,” I replied. “Who is Bloody Mary?”

“You know,” she said, tossing out the words scornfully.

“I know Britney, but I don’t know who you are. Make me understand.”

“BLOODY MARY, BLOODY MARY,” she yelled. Then she dropped her head and looked down at her lap.

When she raised her head about a minute later, her facial expression was once again familiar. Bloody Mary was gone.

Britney looked at me but didn’t make eye contact. She said simply, “I want to go back to my room. I’m sleepy.”

I paused, trying to figure out what to do. Nothing. I had nothing.

“OK, Britney. Let’s go.”

The conversation had lasted less than five minutes and was over. I walked her back to her room. She lay down on the bed and turned toward the wall. Patting her on her shoulder, I left.

As I drove home, I realized I had just witnessed something extraordinary. Two unfamiliar voices spoke to me. I don’t know if Britney was parroting voices she heard in her head or if the voices were part of her dissociative personalities that her abuse had created to help her cope. I will most likely never know. I never saw or heard them again.

Britney had a love/hate relationship with her staff. She had a roommate whom she either considered her best friend or her worst enemy. Britney craved constant drama and attention, sometimes using this to control the situation and get her way. One time, she and her roommate went to Walmart with staff. Britney got upset and refused to get out of the car. After fussing and complaining while staff encouraged her to go into the store just for a few minutes, she suddenly opened the car door and ran as fast as she could. She was a large woman and not particularly agile, but she had a head start on her staff and made it to a nearby street. Running into the middle of the street, she plopped down, and quickly pulled her blouse off over her head.

Cars stopped. Staff couldn't get her to move, and after a few minutes someone called the police. In the meantime, Britney peed in the road and proceeded to slap it with her hands as if she was playing in water.

Cars were still stopped, and occupants watched as police officers, along with staff, attempted to get Britney out of the road. They tried to lift her, by her arms, but failed because she was 250 pounds of dead, floppy weight. They pleaded and tried to reason with her but nothing worked. She sat there for about ten or fifteen minutes, blocking traffic. Then suddenly, without prompting, she got up, walked back to the car and got in. Mission accomplished. No Walmart; they were going home.

It can be challenging to distinguish between bad behavior and mental illness. In my personal experience, many professionals have a harder time making the distinction than daily caregivers. Expertise alone is not enough. If I must choose between the expert's evaluation of behavior and the caregiver's evaluation, I will usually go with the caregiver. Nothing—nothing—takes the place of quantity of time spent with the individual to really know him. Unfortunately, caregivers are usually not involved in developing plans or making decisions. I believe hands-on staff should be part of every planning group and every policy making meeting. They know the clients best.

It is often difficult to know when a client is telling you the truth, when they are lying, or when they are simply confused. Britney, like many other clients I have had, sometimes made things up to get attention. But since she was also schizophrenic, at times her reality was distorted. She had been severely sexually abused when she was a child, and I always wondered if that could have been the reason for her dissociative disorder; a method of coping with the horror she had experienced.

Britney told me on several occasions through the years that she had had a baby and "they" had killed it. The first time she told me this I dismissed it as attention seeking. But later I came to wonder if perhaps when she was young she was given an abortion. She was certainly smart enough to realize what was going on. Perhaps a relative who had abused her just made the results of that abuse go away. Barbara always insisted she was telling the truth, and although she didn't give details, she never backed down from her story. By its very nature, sexual abuse is filled with dark secrets. But we had indicators, red flags along the way. Britney would sometimes self-harm by scratching her arms until they bled, or by inserting various items into her vagina, resulting in injury. Perhaps this was her way of coping, using her voice, long after the fact.

CHAPTER 9

Psychiatric Wards

Psychiatric wards in the United States have come a long way since 1752, when the Quakers first attempted to care for the mentally ill. There were rooms set aside in the basement of a Pennsylvania Hospital with shackles attached to the walls. These were intended to house a small number of mentally ill patients, but the demand was so great that within a year or two a separate ward with more beds was opened next door. In 1814, the Quakers established what they called the "Friend's Asylum." It was run by lay staff rather than medical professionals and focused on what was called moral treatment. The facility was built so patients could take advantage of a secluded, peaceful, country setting with a system of rewards for rational behavior. These included recreation and work opportunities. When restraints were needed, they were used for shorter periods of time. The end goal was to cure the patient by using humane treatment in natural surroundings.

Many hospitals incorporated some of these progressive ideas in their own psychiatric facilities, but they used medical doctors and nurses instead of lay personnel. According to Penn Nursing at the University of Pennsylvania, by the 1870s almost every state had a mental asylum. And the National Institute of Health says that by 1890 every state had at least one public mental institution supported by tax dollars. There have been many changes in mental health treatment through the years; many good, and some not so good.

Deinstitutionalization began in the mid 1950s and continues today. A movement to shut down institutions and move the care of the mentally ill to communities was well-intentioned and worked for some of the residents. But for the severely mentally ill, the movement was generally a failure. We can look around us and see the results.

Many are still institutionalized; but now they are in county jails, state prisons, nursing homes, and on psychiatric hospital wards. These places cannot provide all the support necessary for patients to eventually return to a functioning place in society, and they cost the taxpayer much more than long-term psychiatric institutions. Many remain on the streets or under overpasses and never receive appropriate care. Although outpatient services are often available, many do not receive them due to various reasons: lack of transportation, failure to understand the severity of the need, inability to organize schedules or thoughts, inability to remember appointments or function well enough to seek help when needed.

The reasons behind deinstitutionalizing were varied, but mental health never received adequate funding for the number of people needing the services. And it is true that some who were institutionalized could be better cared for in a community or home setting. Some could be treated on an outpatient basis.

The conditions in some of the state institutions were horrific. Most of us have seen graphic photos of over-medicated patients sitting in a corner, heads tilted sideways, drooling. We have seen the photos of straggled haired, dirty women and unshaven, sloppily dressed men sitting on benches or in chairs; vacant eyes staring into the distance or into their laps. We have seen the occasional photo of someone in a strait jacket, tied to a chair. They touched us and we wanted to stop the hurt. But rather than figure out how to improve the institutions and make them accountable, we closed them down. I understood the severity of the problems. I worked in two of them.

While I was still in college, I worked for Bryce Hospital, then referred to as the State Hospital for the Insane. It first opened shortly before the Civil War in April 1861. Its mission was humane and included treatment and rehabilitation for mental disorders. By the time I arrived there in the 1970s, more than 5,000 patients were housed on the sprawling grounds. But it was underfunded, understaffed, and falling into disrepair even as the numbers of patients increased. I only worked there briefly; my assigned schedule didn't allow me to fulfill other responsibilities. But I was there long enough to see that much improvement was needed. I discovered that this state institution was defending itself against a major lawsuit filed a few years before I arrived, focusing on patient's rights, specifying insufficient staffing, among other issues. The state eventually lost, resulting in the creation of minimum-care standards for mentally ill patients, which other states soon used as a model (Wyatt vs Stickney).

I stayed in the mental health field. I began working at another state institution nearby. It was known as the State School and Hospital for the Mentally Retarded. That is when I discovered my niche: working with people with intellectual and developmental challenges.

Partlow was founded in the early 1920's and, like most similar residential facilities, had never been adequately funded. There was too little focus on rehabilitation or treatment. Poorly trained, overworked orderlies were unable to provide the needed level of care. Being understaffed meant much of the work done was simply custodial. At the time I was employed, there were about 2,500 residential patients. The school and hospital closed in 2011.

My new workplace had been added to the lawsuit a year or so after it was filed. I worked in the campus school, and although we had issues to deal with, for the most part the staff was adequate, caring, and engaged. My biggest concern at that time was the way the school and hospital were used by courts and social services. They sometimes used it as a drop-off place for (mostly) male teenagers who had major behavioral issues—those they considered "juvenile delinquents." Foster parents couldn't handle them, public schools couldn't handle them, and they got kicked out of group homes. So they were sent to this state institution for the mentally challenged even though most of the time they were of average intelligence. Many were street smart, and they were living among patients with much lower cognitive ability. The teenagers took advantage of the more vulnerable, developmentally-challenged people they lived and interacted with, making staff workloads increase.

It was in this school setting that I was first exposed to a lot of new experiences. The classes I taught were made up only of those with an intellectual disability. We worked on living skills. The students learned, most of them, how to write their names, what town they lived in, the days of the week. They practiced identifying colors and shapes and how to politely introduce themselves. We talked a lot about basic hygiene. A *lot.*

Across the hall was an art teacher. The higher functioning students not only learned drawing and painting, but some were able to make projects using leaded glass. We had an occupational therapist on site who worked with specific clients who needed help with their motor skills. We had a gym nearby for physical activities. The school was a happy escape from the dark wards the patients lived on.

But it was also restrictive and structured, neither of which the teens, who had no disabilities, appreciated. They were used to a lot more freedom and didn't like either direction or intervention. It was here I received my first physical threat.

I don't remember the cause of the altercation, but I needed to stop two male teenagers from turning their argument into a fist fight. At the time, I wasn't quite twenty-one years old and was still in college. I had no idea what I was doing when I stepped between them.

The next thing I knew I had been grabbed by one of the guys. With one hand he pulled me back against himself, with the other he held a brick up next to my head. I don't remember being scared. Somehow, I sensed that this wasn't about me. He was using the threat against me to get his would-be assailant to back off. It worked. The other guy didn't want the situation to escalate. Frankie dropped his arm and released me. I don't remember what he did with the brick. Later, I was curious as to where it had come from. It seemed to suddenly appear out of nowhere.

These scuffles were a regular occurrence, although it was rare for any type of weapon to be involved. I did confront a knife once, though. Marcus was stomping down the hall outside of my classroom, upset at something or someone. When I heard his angry tirade, I stepped out of my classroom. Other teachers heard the commotion and came into the hall.

As I approached him, he pulled a knife and threatened me with it. In the south, where I grew up, being given a pocketknife by your daddy or granddaddy was a rite of passage for most twelve-year-olds. But this wasn't a pocketknife. It wasn't a fishing knife either. Since that exhausted my knowledge on knives, I assumed it was a "city" knife, with a different purpose all together.

Here I need to admit something: when in crisis, my normally easily distracted mind slows down to process what is occurring. In retrospect, I think this trait has kept me from showing signs of fear, or from lashing out, or overreacting in a crisis. When I didn't immediately respond, but stood there looking at Marcus curiously, he was puzzled and then started verbally expressing (yelling) what he was upset about. I drew him out and was able to talk him down. He gave me the knife and it was over. From then on, we were friends. Maybe God used my slowness in responding to protect me.

One situation stands out to me from my time in the state institution. I worked in the school, but one day before work I headed to one of the many large buildings on the compound that served as a residential dorm. I wanted to see firsthand what home looked like for my students.

The building I entered had a large common area in the middle, with individual rooms located around the perimeter. Many of the residents were not in the building. Some were out with staff enjoying the sunshine on the grounds, some were involved in various activities or therapies. The ones left inside needed more individualized care and supervision.

Several staff were moving around or through the common area where they were stationed. They were responsible for cleaning, laundry, meals, and general supervision. If something happened to a patient on their watch, the buck stopped with them. They were generally uneducated and earned low wages, way too little for the responsibilities they had.

I quickly glanced around the room and nodded toward a staff member as she walked by carrying a load of laundry. My eyes came to rest on a large structure in the middle of the room. If I remember correctly, it was about 6' × 6' × 6'. I realized I was looking at a large, cube-shaped, metal cage with a small boy inside. He laughed and made incoherent sounds, but no decipherable words. I sensed this was his way of communicating. He was welcoming a visitor.

I walked to the cage. He immediately stuck a small, white hand through and reached out to me, grinning broadly and still babbling. I shook his hand and then held it until he pulled it back and started climbing up the side of the cage. I watched him reach the top and laugh again, pleased to show out for me.

His name was Kenny. He was about four years old and needed a haircut. He was dressed simply in clean shorts and a t-shirt and was barefoot.

One of the staff walked up. She spoke to Kenny first, sounding more like a grandmother than a paid caregiver. He climbed down from the top of the cage and stuck his hand through the bars. While she caressed it, she talked to me.

Kenny had been dropped off by his parents when he was younger due to his profound mental retardation. An average IQ is between 90 and 110; profound MR, as it was known at the time, indicated an IQ of less than 20.

Kenny also had severe attention-deficit/hyperactivity disorder, more commonly known as ADHD. A few years earlier it was known as hyperkinetic impulse disorder. There was not enough staff to give Kenny a one-on-one caregiver all day, needed just to keep him safe. So someone had come up with the idea of a cage. It was deliberately placed in the center of the room so that when staff was limited, he could still interact and be in the middle of all the activity. Kenny could observe both staff and his peers and be a part of the group. Someone would have eyes on him all the time so every need could be addressed.

I hung around for a while, and as others entered or left the building they would stop and greet Kenny. It occurred to me that this was surely on the list of terrible things for which the state was being sued. Seeing Kenny hang off the bars inside a large metal cage must have been a jolt to people touring the facilities, just as it had been for me.

But here are my takeaways.

Kenny was a constant danger to himself and, like a hyperactive two year old, needed to be protected.

There wasn't enough staff to provide one-on-one supervision, but staff was given the responsibility to keep him safe.

Someone came up with a creative solution.

The cage was like a large playpen with a top on it.

It was a thousand times better than physical restraint.

He could still see and interact with everyone who entered or left the ward.

He appeared to be well cared for and happy.

When staffing was adequate, he was taken out of the cage.

Controversial method, yes. But those tasked with protecting Kenny had few resources. If state funding had been sufficient, Kenny could have had a one-on-one caregiver every waking hour. I never blamed the staff. They did the best they could. And at the end of the day, I couldn't come up with a better idea.

Kenny was still laughing and babbling when I left. He had eaten a snack and was once again climbing the bars of the cage. I only saw him one other time. My mother was in town visiting and came to see where I worked. I took her on a tour, including Kenny's ward. She talked and smiled at him through the bars of his cage as I turned to speak with nearby staff. When I turned back around, I noticed she had another small visitor from down the hall who wanted to make friends. Mom was standing totally still and quiet, slightly smiling, looking down at him, as he chewed the buttons off her dress.

In recent years I have made many visits to psychiatric facilities. They are clean, well lit, and modern. They abound with orderlies and professional staff. They are far removed from the large state institutions of an earlier time and are a godsend to many who need treatment. But I have come to realize that state-of-the-art facilities with trained staff cannot *automatically* be considered great places for the mentally ill to be treated. Regardless of whether it is well known, or simply a small community facility, every patient needs an advocate, either family member or friend. People are admitted due to severe mental problems. They are not thinking clearly. New medications or their side effects can also affect thought processes. And if they are intellectually challenged, they may not understand much of what is going on. An advocate who focuses on the patient makes the hospital accountable for proper care.

Brad was a young man with an intellectual disability and schizophrenia, who cycled into psychosis at least annually. Although he was on several psychotropic medications to manage his illness, his medicines had to be adjusted every so often because they stopped working effectively. He would have a psychotic episode resulting in a trip to the ER. After an evaluation, the usual procedure is for the patient to be transferred to the first psych hospital in the area with an open bed. A bed became available at a distinguished hospital half an hour away. I expected exceptional treatment.

As soon as Brad was admitted, I called the psych ward and spoke to his nurse. I gave her a list of the medications and dosages he was currently on, including four psychotropics to manage his mood, anxiety, and schizophrenia. She thanked me and said she was taking notes. I gave her the name and contact info for his regular psychiatrist and asked for the attending to call him so they could work together. Brad was a difficult case.

The next day, I called to check on him. A different nurse answered the phone. When I asked about medication changes, she told me that since they didn't know what medication Brad was on, they discontinued all of them.

This was alarming. Psychotropics, when changed, should be gradually tapered to minimize adverse side effects. Suddenly stopping these types of drugs can lead to greater instability and terrible side effects.

“Oh, no.” I said. “Yesterday I gave the nurse a complete list of all his current medications. She said she would note them in his chart.”

“Well, there is no record of them.”

“Let me give them to you again,” I urged. One by one, I gave her the list of medications and dosages.

“Has any contact been made with his regular psychiatrist?”

“We don’t have that contact info,” she replied.

This, too, had been given the day before. But I gave it to her again.

The next day I called back. “What med changes have been made?” I asked the desk nurse on the ward.

She checked. Nothing updated since yesterday. He was not back on his regular medication.

`Whatttt?? I was more than a little upset at this news. Having dealt with patients on psychotropic drugs, I knew the list of withdrawal symptoms was long and included tremors, muscle pain, nausea, anxiety, and insomnia. I had never seen a psychiatrist suddenly stop an entire group of these types of medications before. And Brad had been on some of these for over ten years.

“Why?” I asked her. “Why did the doc prescribe all new medication?”

"Well, we had no way of knowing what he was currently taking."

"Ma'am," I tried to control my anger, "I called and gave you the complete list, as well as his regular psychiatrist's contact info. Twice."

"I don't have any record of it."

Sigh.

I wish I could say this was the only negative thing that occurred. But a couple of weeks later I was called and told to come pick him up. He was being discharged.

"How has his behavior been?" I asked.

"Good," the nurse told me. "He is no problem at all. He is ready to be discharged."

One thing you learn as a seasoned social worker is to ask specific questions if you want to know what is *really* going on.

"When was his last behavioral incident?"

"Let me look at his chart . . . umm . . . yesterday."

"What did he do?"

"He was involved in an altercation in the cafeteria. He had to be restrained and put in isolation for a couple of hours."

"How many times this week has he needed to be physically restrained?"

"Let me check—three, I think. I know one time we gave him a shot of Haldol to calm him down."

Great, I'm thinking to myself. You just told me he is doing fine.

I refused to pick him up. The result was that several people on his treatment team at the hospital got upset. They weren't used to being questioned and scheduled a meeting a few days later with his conservator, the director of his provider agency, and me. Well, I thought to myself, this should be fun.

As soon as the doctor walked in, I knew she was not happy. She began by telling us that Brad was ready to go home, that he was back to his baseline (his normal functioning before hospitalization). I knew that she had no idea what his baseline *was*. None of us had been contacted to get info on Brad. Communication and cooperation were both big weaknesses in their system.

She continued to talk about medications she was sending him home on. When one of us made a comment, it was dismissed in an arrogant manner. While she was talking, I couldn't help but think that she had only a few years' training in the psych field and she was talking down to us, who combined had well over fifty-years' experience. She insisted he was ready to be discharged. We disagreed.

Then Brad walked in. He looked pretty good, except he had put on a few pounds. Well, he had gained more than a few pounds, but he was smiling. He sat down, saying he was ready to go home. I told him that's what the meeting was about; we were trying to determine if he was ready. He immediately got upset, jumped up, and loudly insisted he was going home *now.* He said he was told he was going home *today*. The doctor said something intended to calm him down, but instead he snapped and lunged toward her. She looked startled and scared. We pulled him back away from her as he continued his cursing and yelling. Suddenly he broke free and ran, still yelling, out of the small room. A nurse appeared at the door, and the doctor quickly instructed her to give him an injection of something. I didn't hear what drug she requested, but I assumed it was probably Haldol. I knew it would quickly take effect and he would sleep for a while. So much for him being ready for discharge.

A couple of weeks later, Brad was ready to go home. This time I knew he was stable, so I went to pick him up. When I walked in, he was standing by the nurse's desk, smiling broadly.

I greeted him, trying not to stare. I didn't recognize the clothes he wore. He had gained so much weight I was shocked. It was like looking at Tim Allen as Santa Clause. I mentioned it to the nurse.

"Oh?" she said. "I can't tell."

"These aren't his clothes," I added. "He is wearing someone else's, probably because his don't fit."

She looked at me as if I were crazy. I started to leave with Brad but turned back.

"Will you please check Brad's chart and see what he weighed when he was admitted thirty days ago?"

Reluctantly, she pulled out his chart. There it was. 162 pounds on admission. Brad was 5'8".

I had another request. I wanted her to weigh him right then, in front of me before we left. On the same scales. I could tell she felt this was an imposition but again she complied.

I knew it. The scales said 193 pounds. He had been in this hospital for thirty days and had gained thirty-one pounds. I was not crazy. The nurse didn't look surprised and had no explanation, no visible curiosity about how Brad had gained that much weight so quickly. She just wanted me to take him and go.

Over the next few days, I talked to Brad about his stay. His favorite part was that he got to eat and drink whenever he wanted. He estimated he was drinking about a dozen bottles of Gatorade per day in addition to all the snacks he wanted. Well, I thought, that explains it. A twenty-ounce bottle of Gatorade has 150 calories. Just his Gatorade would have added around 1800 calories per day every day.

If Brad's doctors and nurses had listened to us, his support team, they would have known he is food and drink obsessed and has no cut-off valve. Without external controls, he will eat and drink until he throws up. I believe the hospital support staff was feeding him to keep his behavior in check, so they didn't have to address it.

As I mentioned previously, Brad had to be hospitalized from time to time to have his medications adjusted. After a two-week stay at a different psychiatric hospital, Brad was discharged with the following summary.

Brad Johnson:

** Weight 189 lbs. (He weighed 158 pounds)

** Anticipated post discharge problems: Noncompliance with medications, relapse on drugs and/or alcohol. (In the ten years I have known him, he has never—not even once—refused to take his medication. He has never used drugs or alcohol.)

** Recommended Solutions: Encouraged to attend Alcoholics Anonymous and/or Narcotics Anonymous. (Again, he has never used drugs or alcohol.)

These were discharge instructions for staff to follow up with at home.

I cannot overstate this: every person who is admitted to a psych ward for any length of time needs a family member or other advocate nearby to assure that best care practices are followed.

CHAPTER 10

Medical Situations

Kofi emigrated with his family from Ghana. At the age of four, he contracted cerebral malaria, and it disrupted the normal processes of his brain, causing severe developmental delay. When I began working with Kofi, he was in his late twenties, profoundly intellectually challenged, and suffering from seizures.

He had come to the United States years earlier with his mother, Wafaa, and three siblings. Their trek was arduous and involved walking through multiple African countries. In addition to wanting a better life for the family, Wafaa's motivation was to get better care for Kofi. He was difficult to control. Having the mind of a toddler and the body of an adult meant there was a need for supervision every single minute of the day. I recall his mother telling me of an incident where Kofi had fallen into a cooking fire when he was young. His face still bore the scars.

Kofi and his family came to the United States when President Obama was in the White House. Wafaa and other family members became US citizens. Through his mother, Kofi applied for and got a social security number, and ultimately received a monthly benefit from Social Security. Due to his severe disabilities, he was placed by the state with a provider agency. They found him a place to live, with a roommate, and staffed the home with someone to care for him around the clock. Medication controlled his seizures most of the time. Kofi was a tall, dark young man with a huge smile. Much needed dental work was completed, and he was happy and handsome. He saw his family often and sometimes went home for the weekend. He especially loved his mama's African cooking. The agency provided the daily supervision he needed, and his staff grew to love him. Over time, they were able to understand a few words that he spoke. Kofi loved music and staff played it often. He would listen, smile, and sway.

Things were going along smoothly when it became time to renew his benefits. His family was working but all they could get were low paying jobs. They couldn't even provide Kofi's basic needs, so it was necessary to see that his social security continued. About this time, the provider agency was contacted by the immigration office. President Trump was now in office and had instituted some new policies. Suddenly, "America" was unfriendly toward immigrants, even legal ones, like Kofi. The questions the immigration office asked sent out red flags. I was asked to become his conservator due to the possibility of future problems and his mother's limited language skills. We decided, due to the uncertainty of new policies and presidential orders, that we would no longer pursue social security benefits. We did not want to run the risk of him being deported. He was like a toddler in a man's body, totally dependent.

I remembered another client, a young woman from Botswana whose family also overcame many obstacles to bring her to this country. She was beautiful; tall, dark, and slender, but obviously mentally disabled. She could not speak but sometimes made loud noises. She walked in a jerky style, sometimes lurching forward. In her home country, people often mistreated her, sometimes spitting on her as she walked down the street with her family.

"People are good, here." her mother told me." They care for Gorata. They don't make fun of her. America is a wonderful country," she said, tearing up as she spoke.

But back to Kofi.

Social security benefits had stopped, but he had to live. For the next three years, the small provider agency with fewer than twenty-five clients paid Kofi's part of the rent and utilities in the home he shared with a roommate. They provided everything he needed to live a decent life and be happy. They received no funds, including reimbursement, from either the state or federal government. They received no donations. Rent, utilities, clothing, toiletries, household cleaning supplies; whatever was needed was supplied out of love. The owner and director of the agency ate the cost. She deeply cared for this sweet young man with the mind of a small child and made sure he had everything he needed. (The state paid for medical and dental care, as well as daily caregivers, and he received food stamps, but everything else came out of her pocket.)

Over time Kofi's health deteriorated. The seizures became more frequent and more severe. If he caught a virus, his body temperature would plummet. Frequent trips were made to the ER, and sometimes he had to be admitted for days or weeks until the crisis passed. No one could figure out exactly what was causing his problems; eventually, they were attributed to the progression of his disease. Kofi had lived much longer than anyone had predicted or expected, not only out of childhood, but into his thirties.

During one hospital admission, his temp dropped to 89°F. (For reference, hypothermia is diagnosed at 95°F.) The medical team used a warming blanket and sent a warmed saline solution coursing through his veins. We prepared for the worst, but Kofi bounced back after a few days. This happened repeatedly, but each time he recuperated. And then one time he didn't. His body organs began shutting down, his temperature dropped even farther, and he lost consciousness. By this time, I had already made end-of-life decisions, having consulted with family members. Now I had to make the difficult decision to move him to hospice. He barely made the move before he passed from this life.

His family wanted him buried back home in Ghana. I had no idea how to go about that, but I knew it would be terribly expensive, and his family had little money.

The state department responsible for the intellectually challenged doesn't pay for their funerals. Social Security writes a check for $255 for my clients, and they are done. Since the average funeral is between $8000 and $10,000 not including burial plot, and a basic cremation is around $1,000, this tiny amount is quite insulting. Our clients are sometimes buried in what used to be called a pauper's field with few in attendance and no service. If you ever attend one, I assure you it will be permanently seared in your mind.

The agency director, the same one who had paid over $40,000 out of her pocket to support Kofi while he was alive, offered to pay for the funeral. The family selected a casket, then worked on an obituary. Kofi had too many siblings to list; I think we stopped at ten. We discovered that his mother was one of several wives that his father married in his native Africa, and there were many half-brothers and sisters, most of whom were still in Ghana. This large family came together and contributed into a common fund to pay to fly Kofi home. They still came up short, but a relative here in the United States borrowed the difference to not only get Kofi back home, but also to fly Wafaa back to Ghana for the funeral and burial of her son. The funeral director worked tirelessly but found no airline willing to fly into a war zone. He persisted and arranged to have a flight into a neighboring country, then to have the body escorted across the border to his waiting kinsman. Accompanied by his mother, Kofi went home.

Kofi received excellent medical care during his many hospitalizations. But sometimes I have run into difficulty getting the same level of care for my intellectually challenged adults as you and I would receive. I remember having to fill in for another caseworker in a rural county in Tennessee. A young woman had just been taken to the ER, and I was called. She was new to me, nonverbal, and gravely ill. Her mother was already at the hospital when I arrived, but I could see she was overwhelmed by the situation. She was confused by the jargon used by the medical staff and wanted to know if her daughter would be OK. It was too soon to know, but I tried to reassure her that Jackie was getting good care and the doctors would figure out what was wrong with her. My confidence was misplaced.

After about twenty-four hours, I was told they were sending Jackie home. She had not improved and was still critical. I headed back to the hospital.

"Did you find out what is wrong with her?" I asked the nurse, who told me they were getting discharge papers ready.

"Well, no, but she was here once before with the same symptoms."

I could tell Jackie was having difficulty breathing and her oxygen stats were not good.

"No," I said firmly. "She is not going home until you figure out what is wrong with her."

"But we are discharging her now," she insisted.

"No," I repeated. "She is not going home today. No one will pick her up. She is too sick to go home. And if you wheel her outside the ER into the loading area to pressure us into taking her home, I will make sure we get a camera crew here and you will see yourself on the news."

A blank stare was all I got.

I asked what options they had tried to help her breathe more easily.

She told me they had thought about intubating her but didn't indicate that was a serious consideration. I sensed she mentioned it more to placate me than a real possibility. She continued to insist she was being discharged, despite them not knowing why she was so ill.

"She stays," I said. "Please try to figure out what is wrong with her."

The next day when I returned to check on Jackie, the hospital social worker told me that the hospitalist was trying to get medical conservatorship over Jackie.

"Why?" I asked. "She has a mother who can make decisions for her."

"Well," the social worker told me, "The doctor said she can't understand enough to make decisions."

I was livid.

"What? Of course she can. She may be uneducated and poor but she's not stupid. I have no trouble communicating with her. That is out of line. Jackie needs no medical conservator. She has her mother, and I will help explain things if I need to."

I had a bad feeling about this. With medical conservatorship the hospital itself would make decisions, including the probability of not treating her at all. And Jackie's mother would have no say.

The hospital social worker looked uncomfortable.

"Alright," she said resignedly. "I will tell the team what you said."

I didn't have to wait long. I was requested to meet with Jackie's medical team.

In the meeting they tried to explain that nothing else needed to be done for Jackie. I pointed out that she was still very sick and no one knew why. Why hadn't a pulmonologist been called in? I didn't understand why they weren't trying harder, running tests, something, anything, to figure out what was wrong. Why did they keep insisting on releasing her? She could die. She probably *would* die.

By now my questioning was starting to annoy the hospitalist, who was obviously in charge.

"You are not family, and the hospital has a social worker. Why are you involved?" she asked me. I could tell I was trying her patience.

"I am her support coordinator, authorized by the state. Jackie is severely disabled and vulnerable, like a young child. She depends on us to take care of her, and that's all I am trying to do. We need to find out what's wrong with her. I don't understand why she is not getting the care she obviously needs."

The hospitalist had had enough from this pushy social worker from the city. I saw the color rise in her cheeks.

"I'll tell you why," she retorted angrily. "Because our resources are limited, and we think they will be better spent on someone else!"

Ohhhh. That's what I suspected. She didn't think my young, female, black client with a poor mother and the mind of a small child was worth saving. I was appalled, but not surprised. I could have reminded her that Medicare paid Jackie's bills, so she wasn't even a charity case for her regional hospital, but I suspected she didn't care. It was about more than money, even more than time. It was about the worth of one of God's small, broken ones.

This story ended well. Since I wouldn't go away, a pulmonologist was called in and diagnosed the recurring respiratory illness. It was treated with medication. A few days later, Jackie was smiling and able to go home.

But I never forgot. I believe in the goodness of most people. And then something like this happens. It makes me angry that a doctor and her team believed this precious girl's life was not worth saving.

CHAPTER 11

Autism up Close and Personal

Two years ago, I was invited by a thirteen-year-old autistic student to eat lunch with him at his middle school. Alex was excited, and quite specific about the details of the upcoming lunch, emphasizing the fact that this was not a regular lunch. This was a Thanksgiving Feast.

We sat at a round table with three other boys and their guests. It didn't take long to figure out that all the boys were on the autism spectrum, although some were higher functioning than others. There was little conversation among the students as they waited to be told it was time to line up to get their food. Those of us who were invited guests included two moms, a grandpa, and me. We introduced ourselves while we were waiting and made small talk. The students ignored us and each other. Social skills were obviously lacking, and the situation was a bit awkward, although not a surprise. This was a special school that focused on those who learned differently.

After trying and failing to get much interaction from the students, I observed them for about fifteen minutes. Then the announcement came to line up and get our food. The event was organized as a potluck with parents and teachers all contributing. The food was plentiful and looked delicious. Each person selected what they wanted to eat, and then we went back to our table.

Alex, sitting next to me, was having a bad sensory day, which is common for kids on the autism spectrum. They can be super sensitive to smells, sounds, and tastes. Textures, in clothing and food, can precipitate a full emotional and physical meltdown. Nothing looked appetizing to him, although he said he was “starving.” He had three items on his plate: mashed potatoes, macaroni and cheese, and green beans, all in small servings. He was concerned about the green beans, afraid they had been tampered with. He thought he saw little specks of some kind of red spice in them. But at least, he told me, there was no gravy on the mashed potatoes. That would have made them inedible. He was tentative, even about what he himself had chosen to eat.

Looking around, I noticed the contrast between the adults’ plates and the students’ plates. It seemed Alex wasn’t the only picky eater. Only one of his friends had a variety of different foods on his plate with normal size servings. We began to eat. The lunchroom was filled with kids of all ages and their guests. Many were happily conversing, and the noise level was high.

The big guy seated across from me stared down at his plate. It was full of meats and veggies that he himself had selected, but he didn't look happy.

"Pizza. I. Want. Pizza." He stated this clearly and firmly to no one in particular.

The adults continued to eat, no one saying a word. His peers and his mother ignored him.

Then a second boy spoke, but softly, to himself. He was also looking down at his plate. "I will be aware of my surroundings."

Again, no one responded. The third boy looked up from his plate, where he was was stabbing food with his fork, and grinned impishly. "I mutilate my food when I don't want to eat it."

He looked around the table but didn't seem perturbed when there was no reaction.

Then I heard a voice in my right ear. It sounded panicky.

"I am overwhelmed," Alex told me. "I can't eat this food."

"Is it too loud in here?" I asked him.

"Yes. Yes. Yes." He replied repetitively.

I took Alex home. Too much stimulation. He had eaten about half of his mashed potatoes, and only a bite of his macaroni and cheese. (It wasn't Kraft. It needed to be Kraft.)

The green beans with the tiny red specks were left undisturbed on his plate.

There are many developmental disorders, but most of us are at least a little familiar with kids on the autism spectrum. That wasn't true thirty years ago. *Autism* is an umbrella term for someone with certain characteristics that fall on the autism spectrum. It comes from the Greek word "autos" meaning "self." The primary focus of the child is inward. They are isolated by the very traits that define the disorder.

Observable symptoms usually manifest themselves during the first two years of life, but an official diagnosis is often withheld until around age four, sometimes later. This can depend on the severity of the symptoms and allows for different rates of child development. There are many resources for an official checklist of criteria for diagnosis, including the Center for Disease Control (CDC) and the DSM-5 (diagnostic manual used by mental health professionals). An official diagnosis of autism spectrum disorder is not made by brain scan, blood work, or any other medical test. It is based on observable behavior by an expert. And although each person on the spectrum shares some of these traits, each person is also unique. Measurable IQ varies widely.

Communication is a big indicator of autism. Speech is usually delayed for someone on the spectrum. I recall one boy that began speaking much later than his peers, then stopped at age nine. He didn't speak for almost two years, then resumed. No one had an explanation. Sometimes speech never comes, and if it does, it usually lacks what we consider normal speech patterns.

As autistic children age it becomes apparent they struggle with concepts, taking language quite literally. They don't understand nuances or inferences. They have difficulty with similes and metaphors. Phrases like "he is a night owl" are confusing. They look at him and see that he is not an owl. So why did you say that? They don't understand colloquialisms or idioms. For example, we understand "penny pincher" to refer to someone who is stingy with his money. Someone with autism may wonder why anyone would pick up a penny and pinch it between their fingers. Same thing with slang terminology. To someone with autism these may sound like a foreign language that has to be interpreted. These concepts that most people just pick up must be learned. Their brains work differently.

Social skills are severely lacking. Even for those on the spectrum who are fully verbal, conversational speech is difficult. They have trouble picking up on everyday cues for appropriate behavior or speech, like facial expressions, gestures, and body language. Normal back and forth conversation is not part of their skill set. They may fail to initiate conversations or initiate one-sided conversation. They may not respond to social interactions at all. As children, they lack imaginative play, and as they get older, they have difficulty making friends.

Lack of flexibility is a marker that exhibits itself in various ways. Repetitive patterns in play, behavior, and food choices can be easily observed. Repetitive motions or speech is common. Routine is super important to their ability to function; therefore, changes are the enemy. Adaptability is a foreign concept. One way this exhibits itself is in rigid thinking. Rules, whether imposed by others or self-imposed, can be the best friend of one who is autistic. They provide security.

Fixated interests are a way of life to most with autism. Those on the spectrum operate at times within a bubble, intensely focused on whatever they are interested in. It becomes an obsession, and they may fixate exclusively on it for years. Or they may focus on it intensely for months, then fixate on something else. From an observer's view, it sometimes appears they are living *within* the object or subject.

Sensory issues are often unmanageable and overwhelming, not only to the person who has them, but to family members trying to help them adapt to some semblance of "normalcy." This characteristic makes life kind of miserable much of the time, both for the autistic person and those around them. Any one of the senses—taste, touch, sight, smell, and sound—can be so stimulating that the autistic person can barely function. There is no way to predict, and thus no way to avoid what will cause sensory overload. If you see an autistic child melt down in public, usually this is the culprit.

I don't want to sound too discouraging, or too negative. A lot of effort and support is needed as they grow and develop, but with patience, consistency, and love much progress can be made. It is important to remember they don't *think* like most of us. We need to focus on their brain differences. Differences are not necessarily deficits. Some are advantages, as we will see later.

Autism is increasing at an alarming rate. In 2002, there was 1 in 150 kids with this diagnosis. By 2010, only eight years later, 1 in 68 kids was diagnosed on the spectrum. In 2021, that figure had increased to 1 in 44 according to the CDC.

The Autism Speaks website (autismspeaks.org) further breaks that last number down. One in twenty-seven boys are identified as autistic and 1 in 116 girls, making boys four times more likely to be diagnosed with autism than girls.

Those are stunning numbers. Even accounting for better screening and increased awareness, we still don't know why this disorder is progressing at such an alarming rate. Limited studies show that both environment and genetics may play a role, but the key word is *may*. Theories abound, but there are no conclusive studies. Since the early 1900s many things have been blamed: inadequate diet, lack of serotonin in the brain, metabolic imbalances, exposure to toxins in the environment, viral infections, and vaccinations, just to name a few. In the 1950s, one of the prevalent theories was that autism was caused by poor parenting, particularly by the mother's coldness and lack of caring. No specific cause has yet been identified by research studies.

I have followed the development of Alex for fifteen years. One of the first indicators we had that something was wrong was when he was less than a year old and avoided eye contact. He seemed happy; just avoided eye contact. As he got older, I watched him play with blocks. Other toddlers would try to stack them, arrange them, or throw them, but Alex would dump them out of the tub on to the floor. One by one he would pick them up and drop them back in the tub. Then he would dump them out again and put them back in the tub one at a time. He would repeat this until he was distracted or the blocks were removed.

When Alex got upset he screamed and had full meltdowns. These looked like tantrums unless you observed more closely. Then you heard the hysterical shrieks and saw the total loss of self-control. He would kick and refuse to look at you; he would scream until he had trouble breathing, sob, and then start shrieking again. These incidents were never brief and could literally go on for thirty minutes. It was scary to see such a small child so overwhelmed by his emotions and feelings and know we were powerless to calm him. I can only imagine how terrifying it was for him.

Alex was an extremely picky eater. There were only a handful of foods he would eat. Around age six, he only ate green things. His dinner plate would have green beans, green peas, edamame, and broccoli. No seasonings. There was only one item he would eat from a restaurant and that was a bean burrito, no onions, made only by Taco Bell. After several disastrous meals resulting in public meltdowns, his family decided to drive through Taco Bell on the way to wherever they planned to eat and buy two burritos, no onions, for Alex. These he would eat at the restaurant with his family. By age ten, his tastes had somewhat broadened, and he ate mostly yellow or white veggies: potatoes, corn, mac and cheese. He could tell while something was cooking whether he could eat it or not. Tastes, smells, and sounds were triggers for meltdowns. We couldn't predict what would overwhelm him.

His family quickly figured out that in most public places, including restaurants, Alex needed noise-canceling headphones. He also needed a distraction from the activity around him, so his family bought him an iPad and put some simple games on it. For years, the only way the family could eat with friends or in a public setting was to plan in advance for Alex's extreme sensitivity to his environment. They bought bean burritos at Taco Bell, they provided noise-canceling headphones, they distracted him with an iPad. It probably appeared to those sitting nearby that he was simply a spoiled brat. They had no idea what Alex and his family were dealing with. But the accommodations worked, mostly, for a time. Then new sensory issues would pop up and changes would have to be made.

I remember sitting with Alex and his mother at church one Sunday. He sat between us on the pew, his small scrawny legs pulled up under him, his arms wrapped around them tightly. He was about six years old and didn't attend often. He looked a little apprehensive. His mom and I were both watching him closely to see if he could handle the experience. Some days were better than others.

The congregation began to sing. I sang out with exuberance, using the upper part of my range. About half-way through the first verse, I looked over at Alex. He still had his legs drawn up under him, but he both hands clapped tightly over his ears, and big tears silently ran down his face. He looked utterly miserable. It took me a minute to realize that I was the problem. That high-pitched soprano voice was too much for his senses. My heart sank.

I stopped singing and leaned over.

"Alex," I whispered. "Is my singing hurting your ears?"

He nodded, tears still falling.

"I am sorry, honey. I didn't know. I won't sing loudly or in a high voice anymore. OK?"

He nodded again.

I dropped my volume and switched to alto. After a little bit, he took his hands off his ears. There was still too much noise around him, but a meltdown had been averted.

The sound that Alex most hated, and still does at age fifteen, was the sound of a smoke alarm going off. He wasn't afraid of fire, but the sound of the alarm immediately put him into sensory overload. It also terrified him.

After trying many different solutions to the problem and failing repeatedly to keep him from shrieking and falling apart, his classroom teachers figured out a solution. They would remove him from the school in advance of a fire drill. Once the alarm stopped, he would go back inside the building with his class.

If the fire alarm went off at home, Alex would grab his ears and scream. His mom had to disconnect all the alarms in his home because he lived in fear of one going off, especially during thunderstorms when there were occasional power surges. This has continued into high school and is indicative of a true phobia. For word lovers, this fear is called igniterroremophobia.

Middle school came and Alex could no longer cope with the educational system. It didn't fit. An individualized plan was developed for him, but it didn't go far enough. He now had to change classes, organize his time and thinking, and he fell apart regularly. To make matters worse, he now had an art class. That meant he had to be creative. He was overwhelmed and hated art class. He referred to his school as Sweet Springs Evil Drawing School.

\But he was good at video games and could focus on them. He also liked board games. He liked the specificity of the rules and would read them and passionately enforce them. No house rules. Alex could only play if all the official rules were followed. He played with a laser focus and was ultra-competitive. He hated to lose, and his dad worked on his poor sportsmanship daily. After a meltdown following a board game Alex had lost, his dad would remind him of proper game etiquette. After years of training, he got used to occasionally losing and remaining calm. He would hold out his hand to the winner, shake it and say, parroting his father, "Congratulations on a game well played."

Alex, like most kids with autism, was complicated. He had many of the defining traits of autism but was also unique. He had a tender heart and asked intelligent questions. He would focus on a topic, subject, or activity, and it became an obsession, sometimes for months or years. Then his interest would fade, and a new interest or obsession would take its place. But he has always been drawn to technology.

Early on, it was simple games he played on the computer or his mom's phone. But at age six, he found a special game.

He was at my house one day, and I allowed him to get on my laptop. It was in the living room where I could keep an eye on him. I assumed he would play the games he was familiar with and went into the kitchen. A few minutes later I walked back by the computer.

"Alex," I asked, "what are you playing?"

"Chess," he replied briskly. His hands were still on the keyboard, and he was looking intensely at the screen.

How cute, I thought to myself. He thinks he's playing chess. Then I looked closer. He *was* playing chess. He was playing against the computer. And *winning.*

"Alex, who taught you to play chess?"

Keeping his eyes on the screen as he contemplated his next move, he responded abruptly, "Nobody. I taught myself."

This obsession lasted only a few months. He regularly beat the computer. It was almost as if he had learned all he could or maybe all he wanted to know. Then he was done and moved on to the next thing.

Around age nine or ten Alex began to be obsessed with moon phases and weather. Waxing crescent, waxing gibbous, waning crescent, waning gibbous moons. Cirrocumulus, nimbostratus, cumulonimbus clouds. Hurricanes, tornadoes, tsunamis, cyclones. He made elaborate chalk drawings of each moon phase, this kid who hated drawing. He followed weather forecasts passionately and kept family and friends updated. He compared weather apps to find the best one. He was almost manic in his research. This lasted for a few years, and then he found another subject in which he could fully immerse himself: couponing. Digital vs. paper, store comparison, clearance bins, filling out surveys to get more money off products, special apps. It was exhausting to watch. But these obsessions made him happy, and his eyes sparkled when he talked about them.

Phobias were still an issue with Alex. Smoke alarms remained primary, with flying insects causing angst. Wasps, of course, and bees, but also June bugs and dragonflies, gnats, and regular flies. He was terrified equally of all of them. Ladybugs, however, were exempted from his fear. He loved them, along with earthworms and snails. Once his aunt saw him gently stroking a snail on the sidewalk with a tiny stick.

Alex did not have some of the symptoms that many on the spectrum have. I have had clients who couldn't walk through a room without touching multiple objects lightly with their forefinger. Some of my autistic clients were expressionless, with what we call a flat affect. They seemed disengaged and showed little emotion except when upset. Some, even as they aged, remained so rigid and inflexible that even changing their schedule slightly caused them great pain. Some were language delayed. Some expressed their frustration by biting or head banging. Sometimes, when he felt overloaded, Alex would hit himself in the head with both hands or bang his head on the floor or wall. These episodes continued as he made his way through his special high school.

With such challenges caused by being on the spectrum, it would be easy to overlook the positives. Alex was eventually diagnosed with Asperger's, which is on the high functioning end of the autism spectrum. His intense focus has paid off as he has gotten older. He is tech savvy and has learned much of what he knows from Internet tutorials and, as he puts it, "I don't know how I know that. I just *know.*"

He has been the computer go-to guy in his schools since he was barely eleven. At times, he can figure out how to repair a computer after the professional tech has failed. Technology is exact, it is detailed, and it involves numbers and mathematics at which Alex excels. He has never had course work or a mentor; he is a natural. He knows the latest models of iPhones and Androids and the pros and cons of each. He understands all the different types of operating systems for phones and computers and has strong opinions on which are the best. For the past several years, he has made elaborate power point presentations for every holiday. He figured out these things on his own.

Another admirable trait I would describe is his sheer doggedness. Alex can remain focused on the end goal when most of us are repeatedly distracted. He has an inclination toward repetitiveness that serves him well in achieving excellence. When he decided to learn Spanish, he checked out all the language apps by rating. He decided on Duolingo and installed an app on his phone to assist him. Every day he would click on the app and practice. He felt out of sorts if he didn't follow his plan.

Even sensitivity to external stimuli can be a positive trait. There are occupations that require minute delineations of smells (like a perfumer) or taste and smell (like a wine sommelier), or sounds. Alex was born with perfect pitch. Studies indicate that between one and five people in every 10,000 have this gift. Researchers are finding that people with autism are more likely to have perfect pitch than the general population, according to Marina Sarris of the Interactive Autism Network at Kennedy Krieger Institute.

Wikipedia defines perfect or absolute pitch as "a rare ability of a person to identify or recreate a given musical note without the benefit of a reference tone." I can't remember when we first realized Alex had this gift, but he was not very old, maybe five. His aunt was a music teacher and had him listen to some basic notes on the piano so he could identify the tones he was hearing. He would wander around the house, listening to sounds that different machines made: the air conditioner, the dishwasher, the clothes dryer. He would listen to the beep of a microwave or a timer. He could tell you what note(s) the police siren was making, or the bird chirping outside his window. It was amazing. And when he called out the note, his aunt would go to the piano and play the note he had identified. He was always right.

There are more famous people with autism spectrum disorder than you might think. Psycom.net lists several: Dan Aykroyd, Albert Einstein, Carl Sagan, and Sir Anthony Hopkins to name just a few. None of these people had an easy time, but they still excelled. They all learned differently than most of the population, but they learned. They focused on their gifts.

Temple Grandin is perhaps the most famous person in the world with autism. She was included in Time Magazine's list of the hundred people who most affect our world. She is a scientist, an author, and has written several books on being autistic. Google her name, find her books, and go to her lectures. You won't get a better understanding of autism anywhere.

CHAPTER 12

The Man-Child Who Tried to Drown Himself

In social work, as in any other profession, we have successes and failures. Jasper was one of my most challenging clients and at the end of the day, I failed.

Jasper was over 6' tall and weighed 140 lbs. soaking wet. He was in his forties and was dually diagnosed with a severe intellectual disability and at least two mental disorders.

Jasper was obsessed with water. And soda and tea and Gatorade and juice, and well, any thin liquid. He drank it rapidly, throwing it to the back of his throat where part of it went directly down his windpipe into his lungs. Ten years before I took over his care, he had been hospitalized for aspiration pneumonia and had a four-inch scar that he told me was a result of an operation on his lungs. Recently, he had been hospitalized again for aspiration pneumonia.

This was not a common disease for someone Jasper's age; it usually affected the elderly and had a mortality rate reaching to 70 percent. Serious stuff. The therapist's plan for health required that we add thickener to everything Jasper drank to help minimize the aspiration. No thin liquids.

I was unaware of the drinking problem when he moved into my home. But I quickly discovered that Jasper had a pee problem. He would have to go to the bathroom literally every forty-five minutes all day. And even then, he would wet himself, sometimes leaving puddles on the floor, despite wearing adult disposable briefs. He peed all day long and got up repeatedly throughout the night to pee. I quickly discovered that he could not go a single hour without wetting himself. And this was adult pee, not kid's pee. Huge quantities. I couldn't figure it out. He seemed to drink a normal amount of liquid so where did this massive amount of water come from?

And the laundry. Huge piles every morning from all the wet bedding: pads, comforters, blankets, sheets, mattress covers, and at least two changes of wet pajamas. Then there were the extra pants, socks, and t-shirts he wore during the day. Sometimes the pee even ran down into his shoes, so they also had to be washed.

Jasper peed everywhere: on the back deck, on the hardwood floor in the living room, on his bedroom carpet, on the kitchen floor, on bathroom tile. He was no respecter of floor coverings.

He peed in the aisle at Walmart. He made puddles on the floor twice while visiting a local hospital. He peed in the sanctuary at church three different times, right after the closing hymn. It ran down his legs onto the carpet. He ruined two mattresses in six months, even with mattress covers and multiple pads. The bed frame itself was rusted where some of the pee ran down the side of the mattress and collected in the rails. In a twenty-four-hour period, Jasper would go to the bathroom sixteen to eighteen times and STILL pee everywhere. It was so bad that we stopped going to restaurants, movies, and the YMCA.

When we did go out, I had to get creative. I knew if Jasper peed in my car, I would never get the smell out. So, I had him pull a large, heavy duty trash bag up around his waist in case he had an accident in my car. If pee soaked through his disposable brief and his pants, the bag would catch the excess. It seemed our whole world revolved around pee prevention, and usually it happened anyway. Constant pee cleanup. Then Jasper slowly began losing weight. We went to see a doctor. One, then another. An ultrasound was done. Blood work was done. Even a CT scan. The psychiatrist checked his medications. But nothing could explain the weight loss or the pee. I was perplexed. How could he release much more liquid than he took in? It just didn't make sense. And then, one day, it did.

I woke in the middle of the night to the sound of running water in the hall bathroom outside my bedroom door. I tapped on the door, opened it, and peeked in. Jasper's long neck was tilted under the sink water faucet; he was slurping and guzzling the water, raising his head every little bit to cough. He was aspirating water with every gulp. I turned off the faucet.

"Why you do that?" he asked angrily. "I need drink water out of faucet."

"No, Jasper, we drink water out of a glass. You are aspirating; it is going down into your lungs and can make you sick."

"NO," he yelled. "I WILL OUT OF FAUCET!"

I learned to sleep lightly and discovered he was drinking copious amounts of water out of the faucet every night. He would get up to pee, drink a lot of water and go back to bed. He would get up to pee again, usually in less than an hour, and drink more water. This went on all night. I tried to reason with him, offered rewards, used every trick I knew, but he wouldn't, or couldn't, stop. I cut the water off in the bathroom. Not long after, I heard him downstairs in the middle of the night. He had grabbed a two-liter bottle of soda and hid in the laundry room. When I opened the door, he was swigging it down like a sailor on his second pint of rum, wiping his mouth on the back of his hand. He hollered, coughed, and spit at me when I took it out of his hand. Well, that didn't work. We hid the soda.

Jasper did not want to drink his liquids with thickener. So he found ways to get water without it—he started drinking out of the toilet.

One night, I awoke to the sound of water and loud hacking. It sounded like someone was taking a shower. At 3:00 am? I called through the bathroom door. No answer. I opened the door and Jasper was standing in the shower, naked, with his mouth turned up to the shower head, water running down his throat. He was gagging and coughing. I turned off the water. He exploded.

"You NOT turn water off!" he yelled, shoving my hand away and reaching to turn it back on. I grabbed his arm and tried to get him to step out of the shower.

"NO," he screamed. I pulled him out of the tub with him fighting me. We both stumbled. I fell to the bathroom floor, and he fell across the toilet, breaking the toilet seat as his long arm reached back toward the faucet handle, trying to turn it back on.

"I HATE YOU," he bellowed. "YOU A MEAN WOMAN."

Jasper's mental or developmental ability had never been told to me, but after living with him for a while, I estimated it to be around three years old in most areas. That explained his language development as shown in his speech patterns. "I hungry," he would say. Or, "Where her book?" "You go mailbox?" he asked me daily.

Jasper understood no number concepts, not even one versus two. He could count to ten but didn't understand the value of a single number. I tried for months to teach him basic numbers, 1 to 10, and a few letters of the alphabet. He could trace symbols on simple worksheets and copy them but simply had no understanding of their meaning. Most people thought Jasper was much higher cognitively than he was due to the fact that he talked a lot. He parroted vocabulary he heard from others, yet he had no understanding of the meaning of many of the words he used (echolalia).

Jasper also had the imagination of a three year old. He looked for rocks in the backyard or at the park, then asked for a paintbrush so he could brush off the dirt "like a scientist." Jasper was convinced he found "old, old, old fossils" that he could sell for a million dollars and get his picture in the paper. On those days he wanted to be a scientist when he grew up.

On another day, he would tell me he wanted to be a clown. "A real clown, with floppy shoes and red nose." He liked to make people laugh, even if he himself didn't always understand the humor.

Jasper loved holidays, at least every one that involved costumes. On the Fourth of July, he wanted to shoot fireworks, wave his flag, and dress up like Uncle Sam. "Stripey suit, tall hat, wig. Long white beard," he requested.

Jasper's obsession with holidays meant his whole world centered around holidays. When we went to the library, he focused on books about them. He only wanted to watch movies or cartoons about holidays, especially Halloween and

Christmas. His topic of conversation was usually holidays, and after a while, everyone around him got tired of the same conversations over and over. His support team decided that Jasper needed to only talk about the holiday coming up next. So, for example, he could read books, watch movies, and talk about Halloween until Halloween was over. Then he needed to leave Halloween behind and start focusing on Thanksgiving. When Thanksgiving passed, he could talk about Christmas. Even with this management tool, he almost slipped into a manic state when he was not limited in the amount of time he could fixate on a holiday. And Jasper still believed in the Easter Bunny and Santa Claus, although he was rational enough to wonder how Santa brought presents to a house with no chimney.

Jasper lied constantly. He sometimes confused reality and fantasy but for the most part knew the difference. He sometimes lied for attention and sometimes told untruths because he believed them. The challenge was to figure out which was which. Jasper told me that his parents both died in a house fire when he was a baby. He gave some details that convinced me he was telling the truth, evoking much sympathy. Months later I discovered that his father shot and killed his mom when he was a toddler. His dad went to prison, and he went to foster care. More than likely, Jasper saw a program on television with a house fire or heard someone relay a story about a house fire. Then he added some details and made the story his own.

He was a mimic. He could copy noises and sounds he heard on audio recordings or movies. He repeated things he heard to make us laugh. And Jasper had his own sense of humor. Once, after getting a super close haircut, he ducked his head, leaned in toward the stylist, and said with a twinkle in his eye, "Rub my head and make a wish!"

Back to the pee problem.

Jasper loved to fill up the cat's bowl with water, and he did it daily. At the beginning, in my naivete and ignorance, I encouraged it. It was a simple chore he could do, and he liked cats. The bowl was in the garage so the cat could access it whenever she was outside. Jasper also liked to bring the mail in every day. Whenever he would walk to the mailbox, he would stop by the garage. And every day he would tell me that the water bowl was empty, and he needed to fill it up. It was a large bowl and the water seemed to disappear rapidly, but we were in the middle of a month of 95 degree plus temperatures, and I had seen another cat hanging around. Over a few weeks, I became suspicious. There was no way that a small cat could drink the amount of water in that large bowl every day. I began checking it myself. Bone dry by late afternoon. I talked to my son about it.

"Do you think," I asked, "that we have a large neighborhood dog drinking up all this water at night?"

"Maybe," he said, "but I haven't seen one coming around."

I hadn't either. I knew we had a skunk that occasionally stopped by, but still. A whole skunk family couldn't drink this much water. This continued for weeks.

One afternoon I checked the cat's water myself. The bowl was empty, but there was water sloshed on the ground around it. Jasper had followed me to the garage and was standing nearby.

"Jasper," I asked, "Have you been pouring out the cat's water?"

"No," he quickly replied, avoiding my eyes.

"Jasper, please look at me." He shuffled his feet uncomfortably and dropped his eyes to the ground.

"Look at my face, please."

Slowly he lifted his eyes.

"Did you pour the cat's water on the ground?"

"Naw. I not, Miss Belinda. I promise."

"Jasper?"

"I not pour on ground."

"Then why does she keep running out of water?"

"Cuz I drink. I drink cat water."

Sometimes I feel clueless. That's too gentle a word. Stupid. I feel stupid.

I am a firm believer in consequences for both good and bad behavior. So, I talked to Jasper.

"Jasper, your constant drinking and peeing has kept us from doing some fun things. It has to stop. I am running my washer constantly. If you pee and soak your bedding, we will go to the laundromat. You can load the washers and dryers, and we will sit there and wait on the clothes to get clean. It won't be fast, but we will wait. We will go as often as we need to, maybe every day. But if we have to go to the laundromat, we won't have time to go to fun places."

"I get drink at laundromat?" he asked, hopefully.

"No, but you can have a drink before we go, and again when we get home."

"But I put money in machine and get drink," he insisted.

"No, we are going to put money in the washing machines and wash the bedding you peed on."

He walked away pouting.

The next morning, his comforter, blanket and bed linens were soaked, as well as three changes of pajamas. He had gotten up during the night because he was wet and changed into dry ones, then wet those, then changed again. So, after breakfast Jasper got a drink with thickener, and we headed back to the laundromat.

After we loaded the wet things into the washers, I took him to the bathroom. Then he sat and stared at the vending machines. Periodically he would beg for coins to put into the drink machine. I tried to distract him.

When it was time to move the clothes from the washers to the dryers, I asked Jasper to help me. He refused. He was still focused on the vending machines. I insisted. Other customers were listening, watching.

I walked over to where he was sitting and took his arm. "Let's finish this up so we can go home, Jasper."

He stood up and followed me. When we got to the middle of the room, he suddenly stopped, then said loudly, "I. WANT. DRINK." He glared at me, not moving. Then he spread his legs apart.

The other customers and I watched in horror as pee ran down his leg and continued onto the floor. Remember, Jasper was an adult, over 6' tall. He stood there, looking at me defiantly. Between his legs was a BIG puddle.

I quickly moved some clean pajamas from the washer to the dryer, thinking they would dry faster than jeans. Jasper stood nearby while I cleaned up the floor. As soon as the pajamas were dry, we went to the bathroom to clean him up as best we could. All the additional wet things now had to be washed, including his socks and tennis shoes. He continued to loudly ask for coins to put into the vending machine for soda. I don't know how many hours we were in the laundromat that day, but we had a customer audience the entire time. I don't know what they were thinking, but I could guess. Why in the world did she bring that man in here? Why can't she control him? Is he crazy? Is she crazy?

OK. That plan didn't work.

We finally got a diagnosis. Psychogenic polydipsia (PPD), also called self-induced water intoxication (SIWI). It sometimes occurs in people diagnosed with schizophrenia. The Internet says it is not terribly uncommon, but neither I, nor Jasper's psychiatrist, nor other mental health professionals I have spoken with have come across a case like his, and collectively we deal with more issues than you can even think up. PPD is a sad disorder because it is not easily managed and causes mental distress to the person suffering from it. It is a true water obsession and is chronic, debilitating, and all-consuming. It cannot be cured.

The median age at death with this diagnosis is fifty-seven. Or to put it in a more staggering way, someone with psychogenic polydipsia has a 75 percent greater chance of dying prematurely compared to a nonpolydipsia patient. (See ncbi.nim.nih.gov>pubmed.)

As I write this, I hear Jasper crying softly in the next room. He has been doing this for about twenty minutes. He will not be comforted. He is upset because he cannot have soda without thickener. The fact that even his body is telling him it is not safe matters little. He will choke, sputter, aspirate, lose his breath, and still beg for more. Every thought leads back to thin liquids. If I mention getting a burger and fries at McDonald's, he is happy until he remembers he cannot have soda with a straw out of the drink machine. Then he doesn't want to go. If I talk about going out to eat at a restaurant, all *he* wants to talk about is how much soda or Gatorade he can have. "NO THICK-IT," he insists. And so, to avoid a scene, and because of the pee problem, we eat at home.

Jasper is now positioned on an alarm pad in front of the TV in his room. I must know his whereabouts every single minute of the day and night. I check on him; he has moved on from crying to pouting.

"But whyyyy can't I have soda," he whines.

I ignore this question, which I answer twenty times a day, and walk over to pick up his laundry basket. I walk downstairs to put another load of clothes in the washer. The alarm goes off, and I hear a loud thud. I drop the basket on the floor and run back up the stairs. Jasper is out of the chair, throwing things around his room. He is no longer pouting but is in full-anger mode. Like a three-year old, he is having a temper tantrum.

"I WILL GET SODA."

I move quickly around his room, picking up various books and other items that are easy for him to grab and throw at me. He curses, calling me a vulgar name. I remove the flat-screen TV from the table so he is not tempted to throw it against the wall or at a window. This is not my first rodeo.

“You can’t stop me,” he says, looking around the room for something else to throw. “I break that window. Go ‘head, call police! I WANT SODA!!”

Instead, I wake up my adult son, and together we take Jasper downstairs and place him on an alarm pad in the middle of the living room, away from furniture and windows. He is furious. I am trying to keep an eye on him and ignore him at the same time. I write on my computer a few feet away, and within about thirty minutes he has settled down. I turn off the alarm pad and escort him to the table for lunch. He has both thickened water and Boost Plus to give him additional calories. Although he eats well, he is still slowly losing weight, and the doctor has prescribed Boost while we try to figure out what is causing the weight loss. Another issue, which we believe is unrelated to the pee output.

CHAPTER 13

Stealing Water

Today was not a good day. As I sit here typing this, I can feel a small knot on my forehead. By bedtime it will be purple. I have a large scrape and bruising on my left wrist and blood spatters on my white pants. But I am more upset than hurt. I had to physically wrestle Jasper away from the bathroom sink again. How can I keep him safe??

I brought him downstairs and sat him at the dining table with some coloring pages and books he liked. He was only about six feet away, right around the corner. I gave him a drink of water with thickener per his prescribed dining plan and walked a few feet into the kitchen to begin making dinner. My son walked into the kitchen and asked where Jasper was.

"In the dining room."

"No, he's not," he said as he headed upstairs.

I ran out of the kitchen and saw the guest bathroom door closed. I knew it would be locked. I broke open the door and there he stood; long neck craned down under the sink faucet. He was coughing water, and I knew he had aspirated. I tried to pull him away from the sink, but he fought me, determined to get one more mouthful of water. I wrestled him out of the bathroom, and somehow in the melee, I got a bump on my forehead. Jasper was furious, and before I knew it, I had received a right hook. His fist went into my eye, and a cut opened below my eyebrow. I pushed him down into a chair (so he no longer had a height advantage) and yelled for my son.

I stood looking down at him, blood dripping down my face, as my son ran down the stairs to help. But Jasper was no longer upset, even after seeing all the blood. He looked satisfied. "There!" he seemed to be saying. "This is what happens when you don't let me drink out of the faucet."

We put Jasper on his alarm pad and after I cleaned up, I finished making dinner.

But he still wanted water.

"Just let me have water," he yelled from the next room. "I don't care if I die. Just leave me alone, and let me drink out of faucet. Pleeease, Miss Belinda."

"We have to keep you safe, Jasper. You know you can have all the water you want with thickener."

"NO," he yelled again. "I DRINK OUT OF FAUCET!"

Jasper thinks about drinking all day long. At night when he goes to bed, he will sometimes lie there, obsessing about drinking out of the faucet. After a little while he can bear it no longer. He will jump out of bed and race to the bathroom as the alarm sounds, hoping he can get there before I do. I can never let down my guard. I am exhausted.

We kept trying to come up with a solution and eventually settled on the alarm pad. We decided to place it on top of his mattress while he slept and in his chair during the day. Whenever he got up, I was alerted and could constantly keep my eyes on him. This worked fairly well; but he was always thinking of some way to distract me so he could, as he put it, "steal water."

One day we were out in the community running errands. Jasper had been patient, and I thought a treat was in order.

"Hey Jasper," I said. "How about pizza for lunch? There's a Little Caesar's up ahead. We can buy pizza and take it home. Would you like that?"

"Yeah," he replied.

I pulled up in front of the store. The pizza would already be cooked so I could pay and return quickly. Since it would take only a couple of minutes, and I could see Jasper from the store window, I let him sit in the van while I went inside. There was no one ahead of me, and the transaction was quick. I headed back to the van.

I opened the front passenger door and placed the pizza on the seat.

"Well, I got it, Jasper," I said. "Doesn't it smell good? Let's go home and eat."

As I was talking, I glanced into the back seat. Jasper's head was tilted back against the headrest and lolled to one side. His face was ashen gray. His eyes were closed, and his arms hung limp from his shoulders. I quickly opened the back door next to him.

"Jasper, Jasper," I spoke urgently as I tried to get a response. What was wrong? He was fine a few minutes ago. He had no history of seizures, but he didn't look like he was having a seizure anyway. He looked dead.

I lightly tapped his cheeks and called his name again. Nothing happened. I lifted his right arm and it dropped limply to his side. I grabbed my phone to call 911, then saw a woman nearby, walking to her car. I yelled at her to call 911, quickly reclined the van seat and started doing CPR. No pulse, no response.

This is not working, Belinda. I was talking to myself. "Keep going. Push."

He's not responding.

Keep up the chest compressions.

But he's dead.

Keep pushing. Don't stop.

After a few minutes I realized a small crowd had gathered, including my son and his manager from Little Caesar's. I could see on their faces they thought doing CPR was futile. They thought he was gone. I was getting tired, and my son took over.

"Mom, this isn't doing anything. I think he's dead."

"Don't stop," I said. "The ambulance should be here in a few minutes."

Still no pulse. Then it was my turn again.

Suddenly, Jasper slightly moved his left arm. I kept pushing, rhythmically, on his chest. A small stream of water dribbled out of the corner of his mouth and ran down his shirt. He slowly opened his eyes and looked at me blankly.

That's when the ambulance arrived. The medics took over, stabilized him, then took him to the ER.

I was puzzled. What was wrong with him? I looked around the car and saw an empty water bottle on the floor next to where his feet had been. Suddenly, I realized what must have happened, and Jasper confirmed it later. He had seen a water bottle in the back of the car while we were running errands. He kept thinking about it, and as soon as I left the car he saw his opportunity. He grabbed and drank it so quickly he totally blocked his airway and almost asphyxiated himself.

On Saturday afternoons during football season, family gathered in the living room and watched SEC football. This Saturday, Jasper wanted to join us. My grandson prepared snacks: black grapes, Chex mix, brownies, and cheese crackers were placed on the large wooden coffee table in the middle of the living room. Jasper enjoyed watching the game and sharing the fun. He had his own bottle of flavored water with thickener. He drank it slowly, glancing over after each sip to see if I was still watching him. I was.

When the game was over, I stood up and started clearing away the leftover food. Jasper wanted to check the mail. As he started toward the front door, I walked with him and stood a few steps inside the door. He continued to the mailbox, and I observed him through the glass to make sure he didn't dash over to the neighbors' house and try to drink out of their garden hose again. I saw him walk to the mailbox and open the flap. Just then I heard a voice behind me. It was my autistic grandson, asking me a question.

I turned around and briefly answered him, then looked back out of the window toward the mailbox. Jasper was gone.

I yelled to my daughter to follow me; Jasper was out of sight. By now she knew the drill well, and we both ran quickly down the front steps. She hollered back over her shoulder and instructed my grandson to grab her cell phone and follow us. Once outside, I called Jasper's name and looked around, but he was nowhere to be seen. I ran to the driveway, and followed it down the incline to the garage, located under the house. I burst through the door but had to stop to let my eyes adjust to the darkness. I looked down, and right inside the door was the cat's water bowl. It was empty. I quickly glanced around the garage.

Back in the far-right hand corner was a shadowy figure, and I ran toward it. It was Jasper, and he had his head turned back, gulping out of a water bottle. As I approached him, he backed up as if to get one more swig of water before I got to him. Even though the open garage door had let in some light, my eyes had still not fully adjusted to the semi-darkness. But I could see his pallor was changing from its normal white to a dull gray. His airway was blocked. I knocked the water bottle out of his hand and grabbed his arm.

My daughter was right behind me, and as he started collapsing to the floor, she grabbed his other arm and together we held him up off the concrete floor. With one hand I began hitting him between his shoulder blades to dislodge the water blocking his windpipe. He weakly fell to his knees, eyes rolling back in his head as I continued to hit him on his back. Finally, he expelled the water, and as he coughed and sputtered, we knew once again we had gotten to him in time. My grandson stood in the doorway with the cell phone in his hand and horror on his face.

The state requires that a report be filed each time a significant negative incident occurs during the care of a client. I had previously filed several incident reports concerning Jasper and water, and this was reportable, so I filed it later that day. Much to my surprise, I was soon notified that an internal investigation was being opened against me for neglect. The only reason I could think of was that Jasper had accessed water without thickener under my watch. Never having had a single black mark against me in decades of social work, it bothered me, and I was instructed to meet a state investigator in a nearby town.

Since I was responsible for Jasper twenty-four hours per day, seven days per week, it would be necessary to take him with me to the interview. The next morning, we headed out early in the van for the meeting. Jasper didn't sit up front with me. I learned the hard way that clients need to ride in the back seat. More than once, I had upset clients try to grab the steering wheel while we were going 70 mph on the interstate.

We had gone less than two miles when Jasper suddenly lunged across the back seat to the other side of the van and grabbed something. I heard the crackle of thin plastic and realized he had found a water bottle. As I tried to get the car onto the shoulder of the road safely, Jasper threw his head back and rapidly gulped it down. As the car screeched to a stop, I jumped out and threw open the back door. Reaching across, I grabbed the bottle, but it was already empty, and Jasper was coughing. I looked around the car. Except for a small bag of toys and a Kleenex box, there was nothing in the back seat. Nothing on the floor. So where did the water bottle come from?

I assumed it must have rolled out from under the seat while I was driving. My young grandson sat on that side of the car when he rode with me, and sometimes had a bottle of water with him. Of course, he had been cautioned repeatedly not to leave anything in the car that Jasper could get, but he must have forgotten.

When I took the bottle away, I realized that it must have been half full or less because of how quickly Jasper drank it down. He was ok; this time he didn't even start turning gray. My frustration spilled over.

"WHY?" I raised my voice. "WHY, Jasper? You could have killed us both! The lady behind me almost rear ended us when I pulled over so suddenly. You have to stop guzzling water!"

"I WILL drink water" he yelled. "I WILL!! He began hitting the car window with his fists.

"Jasper, stop. You're going to break the window."

"I NOT STOP I BREAK THIS WINDOW."

I got back behind the wheel and turned the car around to return home. The investigator would have to wait. My adult son was there, and he might be able to help settle Jasper down. I called him on the phone with Jasper yelling in the background. Trying to make myself heard over the noise, I asked my son to watch for us and come out to the van.

Thomas strode out of the front door as I drove up. Jasper was still upset and glaring at the back of my head. I could see his face in the rear-view mirror. This was not a small child I was entrusted to care for. This was a 6'-tall man with a severe psychiatric illness; one I could not fix. I came to a sudden conclusion: I cannot keep him safe. I have tried and tried, but I cannot keep him safe. The next time, and there will be a next time, he may die.

Thomas got into the car, and I told him we were taking Jasper to the emergency room of a nearby hospital. I didn't know what else to do.

"Good," he said. "You should have done it a long time ago. It's just a matter of time before he kills himself. But you've done all you can do. We all have."

At the ER, I explained Jasper's diagnosis: psychogenic polydipsia, schizophrenia, intellectual disability. I gave the doctor and the nurses details.

"He has to be watched constantly," I told them. "No thin liquids. Only beverages with thickener. No soda because the thickener doesn't dissolve in it. He aspirates, and without intervention he would have died three times in the last two months," I told them. "He has been hospitalized at least twice for aspiration pneumonia, including recently at this very hospital. I cannot overstate how serious this is."

Jasper was placed in the psychiatric unit of the ER under the watch of a hospital sitter and a nearby guard. I explained again to the sitter the importance of him being allowed only liquids with thickener, as well as direct supervision while he drank *anything*.

"Watch him carefully," I repeated. I had noticed a nearby trashcan. "He will try to distract you to sneak discarded drinks out of nearby trash cans. And he may beg and cry for you to get him water or soda. And he cannot go to the bathroom alone. He will drink out of the faucet or toilet."

I stayed until he was settled, and then left to be interviewed by the investigator.

After the interview was completed, I had another incident report to file. Imagine my consternation when I was informed a day or two later that a second investigation for neglect had been opened against me. And then a third was opened. I felt shell-shocked. All three had to do with Jasper's access to water.

He was in the ER for about seventy-two hours. I went to his room a few times to see him and talk with the doc or nursing staff. During this time the state insisted I stay with him, even though I was not allowed to sit in his room, and he had a dedicated hospital staff as well as a security guard outside his door to keep him safe. I sat in the waiting room for hours and hours, doing absolutely nothing for Jasper, but the state required it. And I didn't get paid for those days because the hospital, not I, was responsible for his care. The nonsensical policies of the state at times astound me, but I stayed until bedtime then went home. The next morning I drove back to the hospital to check on Jasper. He had an oxygen tube in his nose.

"Why?" I asked the nurse sitting outside his room. She told me he had complained of not being able to breathe well. On further questioning, the reason came to light. Someone, against my specific instructions, had given him thin liquid (coffee) without thickener, and he aspirated. But she didn't mention that fact until I drew it out of her.

The next day the ER was ready to discharge him.

"We have his things ready," they told me. "You can take him home."

"No. I'm not taking him home."

"What do you mean?"

"I can't keep him safe."

"But he is no longer acute."

"Of course he is. I need to talk to the ER doc."

I wouldn't leave, and finally the ER doc came in. I could tell he didn't want to talk to me. I tried to reason with him, but he just repeated what the nurse had told me.

"He is no longer acute. He doesn't meet our criteria to stay."

"This is a chronic disease. I know. But it is also acute. He can die any day of it. That's why I brought him here. Why is he not going to a psych hospital?"

"Four of them turned him down."

"Why?"

"Inability to provide what he needs."

"Let me get this straight. You can't keep him safe, and the psych hospitals can't keep safe but I need to take him home? I've already told my superiors I can't keep him safe. That's why I brought him here."

"Let me explain, Ms. Mitchell. He cannot remain here because he is no longer acute."

"I understand what you are saying. But it is nonsense. He can die at any time."

The doc just kept repeating the same thing. "He is not acute."

I had to take him home.

When a mentally ill person moves in with me, I can usually expect a honeymoon period of about eight weeks. It lulls me into thinking that things are not as bad as I thought they would be, and I relax a little. Around week nine, things begin to change. The personality that was so sweet initially can now be demanding, often belligerent. Entitlement can rear its ugly head. In a family living situation, the whole family must be considered. The clients are often used to being cared for by support staff who work in shifts and focus exclusively on them.

On a given day, one person's needs may rise to the top over the rest of the group. Perhaps your teenager's car breaks down and you have to take him to school, then work, and then to soccer practice. But that is the very day your intellectually-challenged person wants to go out to eat and to a movie. Or to the pool for a swim. But there is no time today. Those things must wait for another day. Then the sweetness may leave and tantrums start. It is one thing for a two year old to have a tantrum; it is another thing entirely to witness an adult male have a tantrum—throwing things, screaming profanities, threatening to knock you down when you know he can do that very thing.

Before Jasper moved in with us, he got his way by threatening physical aggression. Sometimes he shoved, hit, or pushed his caregiver. Sometimes he would make false accusations against staff. Since an open investigation results in the client being removed from the home, and no pay for the accused for a month, even after they are vindicated, staff will often not report the behavior. Nine dollars per hour for shift staff doesn't lend itself to saving for a rainy day. Every day is a rainy day. And although family providers, like I have been, make well above minimum wage, we also have a lot more responsibility and no break from the madness. And we don't get paid during investigations, either.

Jasper thrived on making staff afraid of him. That didn't go over well in my house. When he moved in, I had two twenty-something-year-old sons still living at home. Once Jasper realized no one was afraid of him, most of the threats stopped. But his water obsession worsened and with it the pee problem.

A little while ago, I went to the mirror and checked my eye. It will leave a scar, but because it borders my eyebrow, it will hardly be noticeable. I wonder how long it takes for a black eye to go away?

CHAPTER 14

Spideyman

Early one morning, right before my alarm went off, my oldest son woke me up.

"Mom," he called loudly from downstairs. I got up, walked out into the hall and looked over the railing, to the living room below. Andrew was looking up at me, an odd expression on his face.

"Mom!" he repeated.

"What's going on?"

"Jasper just knocked on the front door." He was alternately looking at me and the front door.

"What?? He is supposed to be in bed. Let him in."

Andrew walked to the front door and unlocked it. He could see Jasper through the glass standing on the stoop. He opened the door, and Jasper walked in. His pajama pants were ripped up one side to his waist, and the tops of his long skinny feet were scratched and bloody. He didn't look hurt, he looked mad, like a grumpy old rooster.

"How did you get outside?" I asked him.

"I jump out window."

"You WHAT?"

"I jump out window."

I was relieved to see that he wasn't hurt badly. The way our lot slopes down, Jasper's window was two-and-a-half stories high. Fortunately, his fall was partially broken by a seventeen-year-old Rose of Sharon bush growing underneath the window, so he just got minor scrapes and bruises.

"But why?" I wanted to know.

"I Spideyman."

"But why?" I asked again. Silence. I could tell he was thinking of how to answer. Finally, he glared at me.

"Because I want go bathroom."

"Your bedroom is next door to the bathroom, Jasper. That's not why you went out the window. Is this about water?"

He narrowed his eyes. "I. Want. Water."

More glaring and silence, until I took him upstairs for his morning shower and cleaned his cuts with alcohol. He screamed like he was dying. Well, I thought to myself, at least he won't jump out the window again. Alcohol stings.

I was wrong. Four days later, Jasper did it again. Now I had *two* problems: how to keep him from peeing all over everything and how to keep him from jumping out of second-story windows. I assumed state protocols restricted me from putting bars on his window. They would probably consider it both a safety and a rights restriction. And special locks wouldn't work. A young woman I knew just broke the glass and cut herself when someone had locks installed on her windows. I finally settled on a window alarm. Although that wouldn't keep him from "escaping" through the window, it would at least let me know he was no longer in his room, and I could check on his safety. A few days later my neighbor told me Jasper sneaked over to his house and tried to drink out of his water hose. Well, that explained a lot.

As in most organizations, the people making the rules rarely have the personal field experience needed to make sensible, appropriate procedures and policies. And those in the trenches who are fighting these daily battles have no say. But the truth goes even beyond that. There are simply situations where *no one* has a clue what to do—not the psychiatrists, the psychologists, the agency administrators, the behavior analysts, not the medical doctors, not the therapists, not the daily hands-on staff, or even the host family, who usually know them better than anyone else. None of us have a clue. Putting labels on behaviors and classifying them is sometimes as far as we can go. There are sometimes no easy answers, and sometimes no answers at all. We just keep trying.

You can call it persistence or stubbornness, it really makes no difference. In spite of myself, and being regularly reminded of my pitiful limitations, there is still a small, naive part of me that thinks if I just try harder, I can find a solution to every problem. I suspect many social workers and mental health professionals share my struggles to maintain that proper balance between what we *think* we can do, and what we *can* do.

CHAPTER 15

Sunshine and Rufio

Most of this book is filled with challenging problems. After all, social workers aren't needed until some life difficulty arises. But there is a lighter side, a fun side, that I don't want to overlook.

In my years of social work, I have managed caseloads, taught classes, and done contract work. I have provided support for clients who needed a home with a caregiver skilled in certain areas like management of inappropriate behavior and its causes. (I have termed this "therapeutic" care giving.) Although no degree or certification is required, there is a lot of experience and self-education involved. These clients need much more than just their physical needs met. In fact, sometimes they can fully care for their physical needs, but they have issues that require round-the-clock care and supervision, not only for their own safety but the safety of others.

The state provides training in such areas as abuse, neglect, and the rights of those with intellectual and mental disorders. A caregiver may also need training in manual restraint. Crisis Prevention Intervention, which is a method to physically restrain someone who is out of control and may hurt themselves or someone else, is an example of this type of training. A caregiver may have to take a medication administration course, in addition to the standard requirements of CPR and first aid. They need to understand diagnoses and treatments of those they support. In addition, they may work with physical or occupational therapists, nutritionists, speech pathologists, and other specialists in supporting their clients.

The more difficult adult clients are usually in their twenties or early thirties. I have housed some for months or years, trying to help them learn skills needed to live in a more independent, stable environment. Often, they have been thrown out or evicted from other homes because of aggressive behavior. Even though we train, and problem solve, we also need to have fun. Enter Sunshine and Rufio.

Darius had moved in with me only a few weeks earlier, and he was difficult to say the least. He had a reputation as a "runner," taking off whenever he got mad about something. He would stay gone for days at a time. I racked my brain trying to think of some way to help him resolve his frequent anger without running off.

We were out shopping one afternoon and stopped by Tractor Supply to buy a large bag of bird seed. As we walked into the store, we heard chirping. It was spring, and dozens of baby chicks and ducks scurried about under heat lamps, waiting for new homes. Darius and I were both enamored, and twenty minutes later we walked out with a cage, poultry starter, and two baby ducks so tiny they were just little puffs of down. We both giggled all the way home.

Over the next several days we researched ducks. I used to live on a farm, so I knew something about chickens, but nothing about ducks. We discovered that the yellow ball of fluff was a Pekin and was usually eaten when it grew up. Darius was horrified. Of course, we wouldn't do that, I told him. When she was fully grown, we would take her to my mother's farm, since our neighborhood covenant didn't allow any farm animals. Darius decided this duck would be his personal pet, and he would take care of her. He named her Sunshine.

The other ball of fluff was black and white. His breed was called Magpie. Because he had a streak of black hair down the center of his scalp, we called him Rufio, one of the lost boys in the Robin Williams movie *Hook*, based on Peter Pan. Rufio turned out to be the more aggressive of the two, and a single curly feather on his tail confirmed he was a male. He had the most personality and the loudest quack.

Darius took his responsibility to care for the ducks seriously. We had placed the cage in the kitchen to keep the babies warm without a heat lamp, so the bedding had to be changed every day due to the stinky smell. They were messy, too. They would step in their water or food bowls and dump out the contents. Water had to be checked several times a day. At night, we covered the cage with a large towel so they would sleep and feel more secure. Darius checked on those ducklings off and on all day. He talked to them as if they were his baby humans.

The first thing Darius did every morning was go out on the back deck and smoke a cigarette. The second thing he did was get wood chip bedding and clean the duck cage, giving them fresh food and water. He was almost religious in his zeal. I was surprised he had taken on his new role so well. Darius had a new focus, so behavioral incidents were down. The ducks made our home more cheerful, and everyone loved having them around, except for my son's tortoise shell cat. She was not a fan.

One thing we soon learned about ducks was how quickly they grow. In about six weeks they outgrew their cage, and we had to borrow a large dog crate from my daughter to house them. We also learned that the poop smell worsened considerably as they grew. Now the bedding had to be changed twice a day, but Darius didn't complain. And although I helped occasionally, he mostly handled the increased cage cleaning problem on his own. But he had a question which I could tell he was struggling with.

"Miss Belinda," he asked me one morning, "why do the ducks poop all the time? Sometimes they even poop while I am cleaning out their cage."

"I don't know," I told him. "Let's google and see if we can figure it out."

After reading for a bit, I had an answer, at least a partial one. We found out that ducks lack a sphincter muscle. They have no control over their, um, output.

We also learned something else. Ducks like earthworms. After breakfast, Darius would head to the back yard, turning over rocks. When he found a worm, he would triumphantly bring it inside, and feed it to Sunshine. Rufio would get the second worm if he had found an extra one. The Internet informed us that green peas were a treat for ducks, and I would buy bags of green peas from the grocery. The ducks would gobble them up, even frozen. They were eating a lot, including the recommended food from Tractor Supply. They started quacking. As they got bigger and bigger the quacks got louder, especially Rufio's. Now they needed to swim.

We first tried the Jacuzzi in the master bathroom. The ducks loved the water, but it was time consuming to clean the tub out every day. So back to Tractor Supply we went, where we purchased a large, metal stock tank. (I will admit, this was not really for the ducks. I had planned to purchase one a little later for a container vegetable garden. But it was still too early to plant, so we filled it with water for the ducks.)

Every afternoon we took them outside to the back yard. They waddled around a little while before their afternoon swim. Darius was still focused on his Sunshine, and his behavior stayed within normal boundaries. I was elated. This was a win-win.

In the meantime, the ducks kept growing. One morning, Darius asked me to look at Sunshine. He thought something was wrong with her. He was right. She was holding her neck in a funny way, almost like she had slept on it wrong.

"We'll watch her," I told Darius. "Maybe it will be normal by tomorrow."

But it wasn't. Over the next few days, it seemed to worsen. Her neck was bent down and crooked. Back to the Internet for information.

"According to this article," I told Darius, "Her condition is called a wry neck. It happens sometimes."

"What causes it?" He wanted to know.

"The article says it is caused by poor nutrition," I replied. "But that doesn't make sense to me because of her diet. We feed her the recommended staple food. And she gets lots of other foods as well."

Darius was thinking hard. "Sunshine eats peas, and earthworms, and birdseed too," he added.

"Yep. And she eats sliced grapes, dandelion leaves, and cracked corn. I don't understand how it could be nutritional. But that is what the breeder articles say so I guess they are right."

We were both watching the ducks as we were talking. Rufio, although smaller, was the alpha duck in this duo. And since Sunshine had a twisted neck, he took advantage of her handicap and pecked at her repeatedly. Darius scolded Rufio for being a bully.

"Let me see if there is a solution," I said. One blog said that extra vitamins should take care of the problem and recommended Poly-Vi-Sol liquid. I remembered giving that to my kids with a dropper when they were young. It worked. Within a few days, Sunshine's neck straightened, and she was her old self again.

Raising baby ducks was fun. But now they had almost outgrown their large crate. It would soon be time to take them to my mom's house. Darius was not happy, although he had accepted their fate. And as it turned out, they didn't go to Alabama after all. We found a wonderful home for them a few miles away. The woman and her daughter adored ducks and already had about a dozen Pekins, but Rufio was the first Magpie, and we had to explain his temperament. He was fun, but rowdy. As they showed us around, I knew this was the best place we could ever find for them.

Darius didn't say much, but I knew he was devastated. He loved his Sunshine. I didn't think the ducks leaving would be a trigger for his bad behavior to resume, but resume it did, and he was unable to live with me much longer. In my opinion, the ducks allowed us to have a little peace, a little respite, from his normal "acting out." So, we both got a time of relative calm thanks to Rufio and Sunshine.

Depending on the clients, and their specific disabilities, we try to get them involved in all types of extracurricular activities. Bowling is usually a favorite, and we take them to movies, parks, lakes. Most of them love the zoo, and those that are higher functioning often like museums. We take them to places they like to go: church, fairs, plays, and sometimes even a road trip. But we are often limited by finances, as well as behavioral outbursts, and wish we could do more.

One favorite special event that our clients get to be involved in is "Night to Shine." It was started by the Tim Tebow Foundation in 2014 to provide a fun prom experience for special needs kids and adults, fourteen and older. The foundation works with community churches to serve as hosts and provide facilities, volunteers, and everything needed to assure the event is completely free for everyone who attends. They provide evening wear, makeup and hair styling, and escorts, as well as a limousine to drive them up to the red carpet in front of the venue. They exit the limo to loud music and are introduced by an announcer with a microphone. Volunteers escort them inside and spend the evening with them: eating, dancing, and making them feel special. And they get photographs to take home at the end of the evening. For one night, they feel like celebrities. I don't know who enjoys the event more, the clients or the volunteers.

Thank you, Tim Tebow.

CHAPTER 16

Eloping

One of the problem behaviors that some of my clients exhibited is what the state calls "eloping"—just walking off from supervision into the community, usually due to being upset over something. At times this does not lead to other problems, and within a few hours the clients calm themselves down and return home. In those cases, it can be therapeutic. Controlled walking is good just like any exercise would be.

Barry comes to mind; walking relieved his anxiety. He would walk the perimeter of the fence in the backyard until he wore a path in the grass. We would often take long walking trails in nearby parks. On the other hand, Barry would sometimes use walking off to express anger. He would take off and walk aimlessly with no idea where he was going. He might go into a woods if one was nearby. The scary part of this is when he would walk down the middle of the street into oncoming traffic and dare the cars to hit him. As someone responsible for his welfare, it was terrifying to see. He used elopement as a way to manipulate the outcome he wanted—usually, to escape a chore, show his anger if he couldn't go shopping as soon as he wanted to go, or if he got caught telling a lie.

A psychiatrist once told me of an elderly client who, for many years, had walked off when he got upset. Now that he was old, he rarely walked off anymore. But he still slept with his boots on just in case he got the urge.

Some people use walking off for a few hours as a temporary way to cool down. Still others walk off for days, usually as an act of defiance, tired of the necessary controls and restrictions on their lives. Some use it as manipulation.

John walked off about every three months. He would walk around town until he got tired and hungry and some of his anger had dissipated, then he was ready to go home. Usually, his walking off was triggered by something minor. He didn't even have to be that upset. But when he started walking, his pride stepped up and he couldn't go back home. The drama had to play itself out. Many times, eloping was a ploy to get him to a psych ward for a few-days break from his regular routine. At times he would call me before he walked off.

"Miss Belinda," he began. "I need a break. Ron and I aren't getting along." (Ron was his caregiver/best friend/bro, depending on John's mood.)

"What's going on?"

"Well, nothing. But I need a break. I need to go to the psych hospital."

"John, we have talked about this many times. You don't go to a psych hospital to get a break."

He begged. "Just for a few days?"

"No," I responded. "Take a walk around the block or play video games in your room until you calm down. In a few days if you still need a break, I will come get you for the day. You can hang out with me."

Sometimes this worked and he settled down. Other times he hung up on me and walked off.

Since John was street savvy, I wasn't too concerned about something bad happening to him. People usually gave him a wide berth because of his large size, although he once got pepper sprayed twice in the same day by the same woman. But he would walk to some place like Walmart and ask passersby for money or cigarettes. Or he would walk to the nearest emergency room, even if it was ten miles away. He would usually tell them he was thinking about hurting himself because he knew they couldn't turn him away if he expressed what we call *suicidal ideation*. John has never had thoughts of suicide or hurting himself in any way. It was a ruse.

John knew hospital and police protocols well. He knew he would talk to ER doctors first and they would call in mobile crisis. If he gave them a good story, mobile crisis would then refer him to a psych ward for a fuller evaluation. He might have to wait forty-eight hours or so before an empty bed in a psych hospital could be found and he was transferred over. If he was moved to the local mental health institute, they would only keep him a brief time, maybe a day or two, and then discharge him because they realized their services were not needed since he was not having a mental health crisis. But if he ended up in a private hospital, he could be there for weeks.

This scenario, which has played out over and over throughout the years, accomplished exactly what John wanted, a break. He got three or four days, sometimes more, with no responsibilities. He ate lots of snacks, watched a lot of TV, and interacted with new people. They were often easy to manipulate, and he got lots of attention. Then he was ready to go back home.

This type of situation happened way too frequently with the population I worked with. I couldn't control everyone's behavior, but I was John's conservator. As conservator, I could influence *his* behavior. I decided that the next time John finagled his way to an ER, I would get involved.

When he eloped again, his staff followed protocol and contacted both the state and me. I called the ER that John seemed to like the best and told them to be on the lookout for him. I explained who I was and why John would shortly show up for a few days "break." I asked them not to admit him but to call me. He showed up, and they called to let me know. I tried to talk to John on the phone, but he hung up on me.

The nurse talked to him, and one of them called me back. "He said he doesn't want to go home."

"I know, but there is nothing wrong at home. He is just acting out. Please do not admit him. Tell him either his caregiver or I will be there to pick him up him shortly."

Five minutes later she called back. "He said he isn't going home, and he wants to go somewhere else. Is there somewhere else he can go?"

I knew she meant well but she didn't know John and that she was being manipulated.

"No," I said, "He has a nice home and he can go there."

She hung up and a few minutes later called back. "John wants to know if you will rent a hotel room for him."

Now I was getting a little frustrated. How many times had John and I played this game? Groundhog Day all over again.

"Definitely not. No hotel room. He has a home. Well," I said, "on second thought, tell him if he doesn't want to go home and sleep in his own bed, I guess they might have room for him at the rescue mission downtown."

A little while later, John's caregiver was on his way to the ER. John still had a bad attitude, but he had decided to back home. I guess he remembered the night several months earlier when he chose to spend a night at a local homeless shelter. He had run off and called the police to come take him to an ER, but they called me first. There was no big issue; it was the same old behavior. This time my conversation was with the police officers.

"No, he doesn't need an ER, he just wants a break. No, I won't put him up in a hotel; he has a nice home and the support and supervision he requires a few miles from here."

John crawled into the back of the police car.

"I am not going home," he said.

The officers wanted to know what to do, where they should take him. I suggested they tell John he had two choices: home or the downtown mission. John chose the mission, and they took him there and dropped him off. He stayed overnight, and after breakfast the next morning he began walking. He walked all day, bumming cigarettes and money for food. When it got dark, he called. He was ready to come home. His caregiver drove to get him.

Weeks later, he told me he hated spending the night at the mission.

"There were too many people and some of them were not nice," he told me.

"You aren't supposed to like it," I replied. "It's for people who have no home, no place to sleep. You have a warm bed in a nice home. It is not intended for you."

"I don't wanna go back," he told me.

"Good," I said. "Next time you get upset, you can walk it off and go back home."

Just to clarify, I would not allow most of my clients to go to the mission. They are too vulnerable. But at 6' 3" and 270 pounds, and having been incarcerated several times, including once for breaking a man's nose, I wasn't afraid John would be taken advantage of, even with his intellectual disability. He can be intimidating and is street smart. This matter of fact, consistent approach worked with John. The elopements became fewer and fewer. At least for a time.

Hakeem was another runner. High functioning, street smart, and manipulative, he was used to getting what he wanted, especially with women. He was handsome and about the same size as John. Mildly intellectually challenged and in his thirties, he was a real handful. He was at risk because of his defiant behavior. Provider families and other staff refused to work with him after experiencing a few of his escapades. He had been thrown out of several homes and needed a place to live. He had been in jail a few times but not recently, so I thought I would give him a try. Everything went well the first few days while we got to know each other.

Hakeem liked to play video games. When we were home, he spent hours at a time playing. That was fine with me because he had no job. He had a few chores, and we spent about thirty hours each week in the community, but otherwise, playing video games was all he wanted to do. This day, Hakeem had played video games all day except for meal breaks. He had a new racing game and didn't want to stop. He started about 8:30 am. It was now almost midnight, and I asked him to please put it away so we could go to bed.

Letting him stay up on his own was not an option. I was responsible and liable for anything that happened, so I needed to be awake and able to respond quickly to any need or to intervene if something inappropriate was occurring. Also, one of my house rules for clients who lived with me was no naps unless they are sick. Some came to me on sleep medication they had been on for years because previous shift staff (staff that work eight hours and are relieved by someone else) reported to the psychiatrist that the client couldn't sleep. But the reason they couldn't sleep at night is that they napped off and on during the day. My job was to supervise, and I couldn't stay up all night and sleep during the day.

Thus, the rule. This was a family setting. I was responsible 24/7, and I could reasonably know that if someone stays awake during the day they would sleep at night, so the rest of the household, including me, could sleep, too.

Hakeem got argumentative. "You can't tell me what to do," he said.

I reminded him that he agreed to the rule before he moved in with me. I tried to reason with him and explained again why staying up all night was not an option. He became more agitated and started cursing at me. My adult son, who lived with me, heard him and came out of his room to try to calm him down. But Hakeem had had enough. He didn't like rules, he told me. He was going to do what he wanted to do and nobody could stop him. After arguing a little longer, he walked down the stairs and out the front door. It was 1:00 am.

This time he was on the street for three days. After three days he went to an ER, and they sent him to a psych ward for a week. He had been without his medication since he walked off and needed to be stabilized, so that was the best call to make for his safety as well as everyone else's.

Still, I was annoyed. It was not a mental health crisis which caused him to elope; he simply acted out when he couldn't get his way. And when he came home ten days after he left, he was still smoldering with anger. He didn't live with me long. He ran away three times in the first month. He has had many failed placements; no one has figured out how to keep him from running off when he gets angry. Until that issue is solved, he will never have a stable home.

Jerome had been wanting a job for over a year. We didn't really think he could hold down a job but decided to let him try. He made it through two and a half weeks of part time work handling carts at Walmart before he eloped. He got mad because staff asked him to complete the few morning chores he had before going to work at 10:00 am. He refused, argued, then cursed at staff and walked off.

He didn't head to work but to the streets. After a while, police were called to see if they could find him. They found him at GameStop trying to sell his Switch game system. He assured them he would return home within two hours. Then he went off radar. We had no idea where he was.

Early the next morning Jerome woke me up, calling from a neighboring town. He used the phone at a workout gym and called me to say he was tired from being up all night. He was ready to go home.

When he got home, he was without his Switch and his athletic shoes. He was wearing dress shoes. On being questioned, he said that someone had taken his new Switch and his tennis shoes. He said he took a bus to the mission, and they gave him a pair of shoes. Maybe. But I suspect he sold his Switch and bought himself new shoes. With Jerome it was hard to tell. Occasionally, there was truth mixed in with his adventure stories.

We still haven't found an effective way to prevent or manage eloping, but we will keep trying. It is a serious behavior because of the vulnerability of the client, as well as being a potential danger to the community.

CHAPTER 17

To Work or Not to Work

Many of our clients who are diagnosed with intellectual challenges, and often additional mental disorders, have until the last few years attended day centers or sheltered workshops. This allowed them to socialize with others and, for those who lived at home, gave family members a much-needed break. In a good day program, they had supervision and assistance with toileting, eating, and any midday medications that needed to be administered. They learned new social skills and perhaps fine motor skills as well. Most people go to work or school; those with developmental challenges went to the workshop or day center. They had a purpose and structure. That's where they hung out with their friends.

Some day centers had various board games and craft activities. They also provided simple life skill training, like practicing good oral hygiene, or how to write their names, or maybe good nutrition. Occasionally, they would take a field trip into the community. Holidays were celebrated. On Halloween there was always a big costume contest with prizes, and on Christmas, Santa stopped by. Valentines were made and shared on Valentine's Day. One center I know had Fun Fridays with lots of music and karaoke.

For those physically disabled, like Mike, who had cerebral palsy and was in a wheelchair, just being around friends and staff brought him pleasure. He hated weekends because he couldn't go to his program. But when the program bus showed up on Monday morning, he was always waiting, eager to go back. He loved everything about the experience and had a special bond with his bus driver. This was a predictable part of his world that was filled with a lack of predictability.

Those who had the ability to work with special supports in place had the option of attending a sheltered workshop. The workshops would contract with private companies, so they had simple work for the clients to do. The work had to be closely supervised, and many of the clients had to be helped by staff to complete the task. But at the end of the week, each one received a small check based on piece work. Some were faster than others, either due to ability or because they didn't socialize as much, but all focused on the work in front of them. The state paid for the staff as well as for the clients to participate in the program.

The work contract might be as simple as counting out twenty-five screws and putting them into small plastic bags. It might be packing selected food items into boxes for a local food bank, or inflating basketballs that came deflated in plastic bags and readying them for shipping. But the type of work was beside the point. The importance of the workshop was that the client was able to spend supervised time with friends and earn a paycheck. The simple act of taking that small check to the bank and getting it cashed brought them pure joy and a sense of accomplishment. I have seen it over and over.

But the state in its wisdom decided to do away with these programs in favor of "real" employment opportunities. On the surface this sounded like a great idea, except to the families and agencies that provided daily support of these individuals. What I personally observed was disheartening. First, there was nothing planned to take the place of the day programs. So people like Mike had no place to go during the day. In addition, the state required many of those they fully supported to be out in the community thirty hours per week, but where? They had little money, if any, to spend for outside activities, and as a result, many spent endless hours sitting in a park somewhere or riding around in a car several days a week with only staff for company, just to meet the community day policy of the state.

Those who lived at home were no better off. Their families lost the break they depended on. They could tell you how difficult it is to take care of an intellectually challenged or mentally ill adult every day, all day. It was exhausting. I have yet to speak to a family who wasn't confused and upset by decisions by their states to shut down the day programs and sheltered workshops.

The reasons shutting down these opportunities for the mentally challenged doesn't work are varied. But at the top of the list are the traits and abilities of those the state wants to place in "real" jobs.

Take Cal, for example. He is articulate and presents himself well. He wants a job, badly, as he will often tell you. He is physically capable of working a simple job, like bussing tables at McDonald's. But he is intellectually challenged and developmentally delayed. He is more than a bit lazy. He may look like an adult and talk like an adult, but his development is that of an eight-year-old boy.

He will work for a half hour at sloth speed, then want a cigarette break. When it is explained to him that he has a break coming later, it upsets him. He wants to smoke NOW. So, he will put down his wiping cloth and walk outside. After the smoke break, he may work another twenty minutes, slowly, with no urgency or attention to detail. Now he is given a broom and asked to sweep the floor. He is shown how to sweep the floor and where to place the broom and dustpan when he is through. He begins.

The manager said to sweep the front, but only when there are no customers standing there. When the manager leaves, Cal decides he can just sweep *around* the people that are there and asks them to move over. The manager notices, comes back to Cal, and reminds him of his instructions. Now Cal will argue with him, because it is important to him to do it his way. These incidents continue and the manager keeps being pulled away from other duties. Now he is getting a little frustrated at Cal and insists he follow directions if he wants a job. Cal gets upset and needs another cigarette break. It has now been twenty minutes and no work has been done, even though Cal is physically able to do the job. Oh, and another thing: a job coach hired and paid by the state has been on the scene and involved the whole time to help make Cal "employable."

The employer, because he is a nice guy and the government sometimes offers incentives to businesses if they hire people from certain disability groups, gives Cal another chance. The job coach takes Cal aside and again talks him through the importance of following directions, listening to the boss, and working steadily. Cal picks up the broom. He starts in the back, where there are no customers. So far, so good. He sweeps for ten minutes, and the boss asks him to buss a few tables. As he busses tables, Cal cleans off leftover french fries. It reminds him he is hungry; but his break is still an hour away. No matter, he props his broom against the wall and tells his job coach it is time to eat. Coach tries to keep him on task but to no avail. He argues loudly. Customers turn to watch. The manager comes out.

"Sorry, Cal. This isn't going to work out."

"Aw, man," Cal responds. "But I really want a job. It's not fair!"

He leaves with his job coach, telling anyone who will listen that the manager was unfair to him, and he didn't do anything wrong. In a few weeks he finds another job, this time at Walmart. Same type of scenario. He gets fired, never having worked a four-hour shift. The state's vocational rehab department reevaluates Cal and reports that he *can* work in the community. The state hires a new job coach to keep him on task. But it doesn't matter. Cal cannot hold down a job, although he has been assessed and the state says he can. He doesn't have the basic set of skills needed: the willingness to follow directions, to work steadily (even with supports), and to control his impulses. Wanting a job and being able to communicate with others are necessary, but in no job are these items alone enough to keep someone employed. And to be blunt, many of our intellectually challenged adults don't really want a job, because they don't like to work. Like children, they just want a paycheck.

I have seen this type of situation play out repeatedly with different clients. Cal did not have the developmental ability to work in a public setting. However, in a sheltered workshop he worked at his own pace and got paid accordingly. In my experience, most of those with intellectual or developmental challenges who were employable in public businesses were already employed. There was no need to shut down the day workshops.

In our local supermarkets and other businesses, I have seen disabled individuals working and doing adequate, sometimes excellent, work for pay. Some have been working for many years. Kudos to these businesses who saw the value of work and gave them a chance. But let's get real; there are also those who are only able to work because other employees have been willing to pick up the slack. They assist or actually do the job when our clients are unable to complete an assigned task due to lack of ability and/or unwillingness.

Everyone needs opportunities to work, but these opportunities must be within our clients' abilities. When we try to place them in jobs they cannot handle, they fail. And the employer will be much slower to hire someone with a mental disability the next time because the first hire caused more problems than it solved.

In my opinion, rather than eliminate the day programs and workshops, we should be innovative and come up with new ways to support clients during the day that provide work, social opportunities, and ways to contribute back as they are able. Farm-based options like learning to grow their own vegetables or care for animals, like chickens, goats, or sheep, would be an excellent activity. It would develop responsibility as they learned new skills that could lead them to other types of meaningful work.

Cal sits at home much of the day playing video games, because there is no sheltered workshop or training program for him to participate in. When he wants a little extra money, he sneaks away from home and staff to steal, or to panhandle, approaching strangers on the street. Or he walks to the pawn shop where he may pawn his game system. Of course, in a few days he wants it back, but he has already spent the money he got for it. Now he has no money *and* no game system. He has few places to go during the day and cannot keep a job due to his lack of basic work skills or his cognitive ability and/or mental disorder. He needs to be in a sheltered workshop where he can do simple piece work at his own pace, make a small check, and spend time with his friends. Let's improve them and bring them back.

Chapter 18

Schizophrenia

Schizophrenia was first described by doctors as far back as Hippocrates around 500 BC. It is found in every culture in the world, primitive as well as developed.

The word *schizophrenia* comes from two Greek words that mean "split mind." The term was first used by Swiss doctor Eugen Bleuler around 1908. It is a chronic and disabling disease characterized by acute behavioral episodes and disturbed thinking, resulting in inappropriate responses to one's surroundings. There is no cure or prevention method, so the disease requires lifelong treatment, according to the Mayo Clinic.

Schizophrenia doesn't seem to have a single cause, but rather appears to be a combination of genetic, environmental, biochemical, and developmental factors. This makes it difficult to either avoid or predict.

Among experts in the field there are many debates about the disease, its origins, its prognosis, and its treatment. I am not an expert, just a mental health professional sharing my observations and insights based on what I have actually seen in my work. The symptoms listed below are not intended to be a comprehensive list, but the most observable symptoms in those with whom I have worked.

Delusions. These can take many forms. For example, they can be persecutory—my teacher is trying to kill me. They may be paranoid—the Chinese are watching me through my television, or my boss is trying to poison me. Sometimes the delusions have to do with identity—I am Jesus Christ, or my daughter is the child of the devil.

Hallucinations. Auditory is the most common. The person hears voices in his head, either talking to each other or to himself. In my experience, these voices can sometimes be neutral, but they are never good or encouraging to the person hearing them. Often they communicate bad thoughts or instructions to the hearer. I remember a young man telling me the people in his head kept telling him to die, die, die over and over. Hallucinations can also be visual, like seeing things that aren't there, or seeing distorted images. For example, the person may see green aliens coming out of the toilet.

But it is important to know that if someone hallucinates, it doesn't necessarily mean they have schizophrenia. Some medications can cause hallucinations, even though they are not listed on the label as a possible side effect. My son, who was eleven at the time, woke up during the night and screamed out. I ran into his room to find him sitting up in his bed, terrified. As I approached, he yelled at me to get back. I stopped where I was and asked him what was wrong. He kept saying he didn't know. Then he said he was seeing things. I asked him to describe to me what he was seeing.

"Tiny heads on normal-sized bodies." His voice was quivering with fear. I wanted to hear it again.

"Andrew, tell me exactly what you see." I tried not to show *my* fear.

"You and Dad, Mom. You have tiny heads, but your bodies are normal sized!"

First thing the next morning I made an appointment at Vanderbilt with a psychologist.

I took Andrew, and he talked to the psychologist alone. Afterward, the psychologist called me aside and told me that Andrew was troubled, and he urged me to set up counseling sessions immediately.

I was confused. I had never seen any indication that my son was troubled. He was happy, active, friendly, and curious; in other words, a normal eleven year old. I didn't immediately set up counseling but decided to wait and observe him for a while.

About a week later I was talking to a friend on the phone, who also happened to be our family practitioner. I don't remember what the call was about, but at some point I mentioned Andrew's strange hallucination. She immediately asked me what medications he was on.

"Nothing," I replied. "He's not on anything."

"Think, Belinda," she insisted. "What has he taken recently?"

"He hasn't been sick," I replied. "So he has had no medicine . . ."—then I remembered—"except Dimetapp for his allergies."

"That's the problem," she told me. "Dimetapp can cause hallucinations in some kids. Whatever you do, don't give him anymore."

I was stunned. Andrew was child number four and all my kids had allergies. Dimetapp had been a go-to for many years. I had no idea that hallucinations could be a possible side effect. He never took another dose. And he never hallucinated again.

But back to schizophrenia symptoms.

Thought insertion. God, the Russians, the FBI put thoughts in my head to control me. An alien has taken over my body and makes me say things I don't want to say.

Flattened affect. A person's speech lacks energy or warmth. Her face may be emotionless. She may speak in a type of monotone voice, maybe even slightly robotic. Sometimes this is also seen in those with autism.

Avolition. The person may sit in one place for a long time doing nothing. There is no interest in activity but instead has a lack of motivation or ability to begin or complete a task. Conversations may be fragmented with little emotion. Enjoyment from life is missing.

The primary treatment for schizophrenia is medication. Some therapies and supports may wrap around the medication but they are secondary treatments. Adherence to prescribed medication is the single most important component for successful long-term management of the disease. Even with careful adherence, the medication must be managed and adjusted or changed as needed. Regular psychiatric care is essential.

During acute psychotic episodes the patient is usually hospitalized for medication management until he returns to his stable baseline. This prevents the patients from harming themselves or someone else. These episodes cannot be ignored. This is not only a health issue but a safety issue for both the person suffering from the disorder and those around him.

A psychotic episode is usually preceded by warning signs. The indicators may include angry outbursts, loss of attention to grooming, muttering to oneself or to the voices in one's head, extreme irritability over insignificant things, challenging authority, cursing, throwing, breaking things, or slamming doors, unusual or inappropriate laughter, or intense mood swings. Each individual exhibits his own warning signs. Family or caregiver must be closely attuned to the specific idiosyncrasies of the person in order to know when an acute episode is imminent.

Schizophrenia is usually diagnosed in the late teens to early thirties and tends to emerge a few years earlier in males than females, according to the National Institute of Mental Health (2018). Generally, the incidence of schizophrenia is two to three times more prevalent in males than females, according to PubMed. About half of those diagnosed have another mental disorder such as depression, or an anxiety disorder such as obsessive-compulsive disorder (OCD).

The National Alliance on Mental Illness (NAMI) says schizophrenia affects about two million people in the United States (1998). While that number seems high, it is less than 1 percent of the population. The treatment success rate is 60 percent. *While under treatment* those with schizophrenia are no more prone to violence than the general population. However, the lifetime risk of suicide is 5 to 8 percent. This can be compared to the suicide risk in people with no mental disorders, which is 0.3 percent according to the Lundby Study (1947–1997).

Individuals often have trouble keeping a job and caring for their daily needs. They rely on family and friends to generally help them navigate through life. Relationships are difficult. Family, friends, and community support are critical.

Famous people with schizophrenia include musician Syd Barrett, founder of Pink Floyd; Zelda Fitzgerald, wife of famous author F. Scott Fitzgerald; Eduard Einstein, second son of Albert Einstein; Peter Green, musician and founder of Fleetwood Mac; Vincent Van Gogh, and Brian Wilson, member of the Beach Boys. There are also many others.

I want to tell you about one.

Lucas.

CHAPTER 19

The Most Popular Boy

Lucas can be charming, with a big toothy smile. He comes across as naive, but this is actually a symptom of his autism, which causes developmental delays. He is intellectually challenged and has been diagnosed with schizophrenia. He is in his mid-twenties. The first time I met him I was totally taken by this young man who looked much younger than his eighteen years.

Lucas was outside, so his family caregiver and I sat in lawn chairs and watched him while we talked. Lucas was walking around with a pad and pencil, totally engrossed in his writing, but he seemed to be having some difficulty. After a few minutes, he walked over to where I was sitting and shoved the tablet and pencil under my nose.

"Write this down," he said with no introduction.

"What do you want me to write?"

"Write this: I AM THE MOST POPULAR BOY. In big letters."

I did as I was instructed and handed the paper back.

"Thank you," he said politely and walked away toward the road.

"What was that about?" I asked his foster mom. My eyes followed him as he stopped next to the road and held up his sign. She smiled.

"Someone at school told him that girls like popular boys, and he wants to make sure that any girls passing by in cars know that he is the *most* popular."

Over time, I learned that Lucas had three half-brothers—same mom, different dads. Both parents were HIV positive due to drug use. His dad was in prison, and his mom died of a drug overdose. His maternal grandmother kept the boys until she could no longer handle them. One of his brothers was mentally ill, and another had AIDS.

Lucas was eighteen months old when the state placed him in foster care. Over the next few years, there were two adoptive families that wanted Lucas, but each stay was brief. He screamed, ate with his hands, and threw food while at the table. He was in and out of foster homes until age five when he was noticed by a worker at the psychiatric hospital where he had been placed for treatment. She felt so much compassion for this little boy that although she was single, she adopted him.

With the help of her parents, Ellie began the difficult journey of giving Lucas stability and helping him grow developmentally. Lucas was already, at age five, extraordinarily manipulative. She began teaching him to eat with a fork or spoon and not to erupt at the table. She worked to stop him from throwing things, making threats, trying to hurt people.

Ellie tried everything she knew to manage and change Lucas's behavior. She explored different therapies, adjusted his diet, gave him special vitamins. She even considered shock therapy. All the psychiatrist could do was prescribe medication, which didn't work very well. She had no time to date, and girlfriends eventually stopped coming around because they were afraid of Lucas. He would bite them and threaten to cut their throats. He talked, as his grandma described it, "devil talk." He would say the devil was nearby and laugh to himself. Around age nine, he suddenly stopped talking. He was mute for about twenty months, then resumed talking as suddenly as he had stopped. No one knows why.

Lucas told his adoptive family stories of being duct taped to a chair by a foster mom and having his head dunked in toilets by older kids due to "acting up." His grandma thought he fabricated them. He was easily influenced by what he saw and heard, so it was possible that the incidents he described never happened at all.

His behavior didn't improve much as he got older. He heard voices in his head, and they kept him agitated. There was a female voice that he became obsessed with and wanted to marry. He wouldn't let the topic go; he threw fits and threatened his mom. Eventually, Ellie gave in and performed a "marriage ceremony" between Lucas and his auditory hallucination. He settled down a bit, but it was temporary. On several occasions he attempted to choke her, leaving a ring of bruises around her neck. Eventually, these attacks resulted in Lucas being removed from his home and once again made a ward of the state.

Lucas was in and out of mental health institutions during his childhood. Because of his double presentation, conflicts sometimes arose between his mom and the medical staff. He would present himself one way to the psychiatric team, and a different way to others, both at home and in the community. One facility in Texas accused Ellie of Munchausen syndrome by proxy (now known by the term *factitious disorder imposed on another*). They believed Ellie herself was mentally ill and making up stories about Lucas, giving him symptoms that didn't really exist. She had to go to court to defend herself. The hospital made a grave mistake in filing the petition against her. She had plenty of indisputable proof of Lucas's disturbing behavior.

Much as an actor perfects his craft, time and practice can make even someone with an intellectual disability quite accomplished at eliciting sympathy. Sometimes they may present as pitiful, ignorant, and vulnerable when they are striking a pose for a specific end goal. Lucas fools most people who meet him casually. On one occasion during a commitment hearing, Lucas was so convincing that the judge came down off the bench, tears in her eyes, to give him a hug. "I am so sorry," she said, "you shouldn't have to live this way."

She had no way of knowing she had just been conned. No one present at the hearing had more than a casual acquaintance with Lucas. No caregiver, family member, conservator, or social worker who knew him was asked to this impromptu hearing. So, seizing his opportunity, Lucas told her he was upset and acting out because his things had been taken away. He didn't want to live at his house anymore because the people who cared for him were *mean.* He meant me.

He told a partial truth. Things *had* been taken away. And some of them he would never get back. But what he *didn't* say was that based on his psychiatrist's recommendation, his state support team took away things that were hurting him and others. His psychiatrist had ordered that all media and items depicting evil characters be restricted because he took on their characteristics and imitated them. This meant he lost his comic books, his DVDs, his toys, and games that depicted evil villains. He could no longer watch a movie with an evil character or check out certain library books. TV shows had to be monitored for appropriateness. It was a rights restriction necessitated by his violent, aggressive behavior. Someone familiar with Lucas could have told the judge that. She never asked.

Also, there were some things taken away temporarily by me. If Lucas got angry and threw his hand-held video game system, or a book, or a shoe, or anything else at me, I kept it for a while until he fully calmed down. Lucas thought this was cruel and unjust.

"You are too harsh on me," he would loudly complain.

For a long time people with mental disabilities had no rights. That has changed, thankfully. But sometimes I believe the pendulum has swung too far the other way. We have taught those with mental challenges how to advocate for themselves, and indeed we should have. But in my world of intellectual disabilities and mental health, we have often gone beyond equal rights. Many of our higher functioning clients have been so well taught about their rights that they use it to their advantage over others.

We often run interference, blocking them from natural consequences of their behavior, so they remain stunted in their emotional and developmental growth. Lucas feels entitled. He thinks natural consequences are cruel. He thinks he is free to destroy things when he gets angry, but then expects you to buy him new ones. He wants to pee in his bed, because he doesn't want to get up and walk to the bathroom, but he doesn't want to do his own laundry. He wants to eat until he throws up, but he doesn't want to get fat. He fully understands the concept, but he believes that although natural consequences apply to everyone else, he should be exempt. Because he is special.

Expectations of those with intellectual disabilities are often lower than needed to foster more independence. When Lucas moved in with me, he was twenty-one years old and didn't like stairs. Our house was on a hill, with a two-story deck on the back, and stairs reaching down to the sloping yard. He had accessed the back yard by going down the driveway and was walking around the perimeter of the yard. I stepped out of the kitchen door onto the upper deck and called him to come inside for dinner. I waited at the top of the steps. Lucas got down on all fours and started climbing up the steps. I was appalled. He had no physical disability.

"Lucas," I called out. He looked up at me.

"What are you doing?"

"Coming upstairs."

"But you're crawling."

"I can't walk up. I'm afraid."

I took the presumptive close.

"Of course you can."

I walked down and stood on the step above him. "Stand up and hold on to the rail on each side."

"I can't."

"Yes, you can. You are a grown man."

I leaned over and helped him stand up. I placed his hands on the rails, first the left, then the right. He slowly straightened to an upright position.

"Now follow me up," I said. "Slowly. One step at a time."

He did. When he reached the top of the stairs, a big smile spread over his face. "I did it," he said proudly.

"Yep. I knew you could."

Then we walked inside.

He practiced slowly walking up and down for the next few days. Before long, he literally bounded up and down those steps.

Expectations had also been low concerning Lucas's grooming abilities. His support plan said that he was unable to button his shirts, and staff must do it for him. Huh? That didn't fit with what I had observed. I suspected he didn't button his own shirts because when he was young it was done for him, and, as he aged, he was never given the responsibility. He was quite accomplished at having others do things for him. So, we had a talk. I explained that I was there to help him do only what he could not do for himself. I was not his maid. Adults buttoned their own clothes. I guided him through the first two times, step by step. He caught on quickly, and it was never mentioned again.

When Lucas got angry, he liked to break things: mirrors, pencils, televisions, furniture, pretty much whatever was nearby. He would kick things, hit, or throw things. We taught natural consequences: if you break something deliberately, you do without. I will not pay to replace it. If you deliberately pee in your bed, you will have to use your spending money to take your clothes to the laundromat. (This natural consequence had to be approved by a Human Rights Committee. But it worked.)

As the months wore on, the property destruction grew less and less, and Lucas stopped peeing in his bed. I have always believed that independence can only be achieved if we learn by trial and error with natural consequences. Unfortunately, the organizations that supervise care for many of these higher-functioning clients believe it is inhumane to expect of them what we expect of others (based on their abilities, of course), and our state training lays the foundation for this concept. While I believe it is cruel to expect things from people of which they are incapable, I also believe it is cruel to expect less than they can accomplish and thereby stunt their growth. My job, *our* job, is to help them become more independent and encourage personal growth so they can more fully be part of their local community.

When outside his home in the community, Lucas had to remain "in line of sight." This was difficult for his caregiver because he wanted to wander off, sometimes, looking for random females. He would approach them, say something inappropriate, invade their personal space, and make them feel uncomfortable. If he became upset while in a store, he might glare at no one in particular and rudely push past others. He would shove children out of his way if they were in his path. He could not push a grocery cart in a store, because when he got upset, he might use it as a weapon to run into a total stranger or to block a particular food section from other customers.

He was so rude and argumentative on occasion that a nearby caregiver was all that kept him from being removed from a store by security. This improved after I took him and went home a couple of times, leaving a half-full shopping cart behind us. He didn't like leaving the grocery store without special food items he had selected.

Since Lucas is on the autism spectrum, intellectually challenged, and has schizophrenia, determining the cause of his behavioral incidents can be quite challenging. Those who are providing one-on-one care, as well as doctors who prescribe medication, must decipher specific behaviors and put them into the correct box to support him in an effective way. Various therapies can be useful, and medication is often critical, but common sense is a necessity.

Lucas cannot have too much alone time. While everyone needs private time, this often presents a problem for someone with schizophrenia. Less outside interaction with his environment leads to more interaction inside his own head. The voices increase dramatically when his mind is not actively engaged elsewhere, which leads to full psychotic episodes. Diversions such as reading, watching TV, playing video games, doing simple chores, or working on a puzzle can sometimes make the voices recede into the background. Their effect on Lucas is then more like a quiet whisper rather than a loud, obnoxious voice demanding immediate attention.

When he first arrived at my home, I noticed that most of the time when we were in the car, Lucas would sit with his head down, staring into his lap. He withdrew from the reality around him and lived in his own space with his voices. So, I made a game of observation. For every fifteen minutes or longer of travel time, Lucas was to notice five interesting things outside the car. When we returned home, he was to list them on a sheet of paper. He didn't like this activity, so I tied it to rewards, usually special food or candy treats.

This worked for a while; then I noticed he had reverted to riding with his head down. When he got home and made his list, he would just recall what he had seen on a previous trip. Lucas didn't like to live in the moment; it interrupted his internal life. But with time, his observation skills improved, and he eventually learned to enjoy looking out his window. This resulted in fewer voice episodes and fewer outbursts.

Although mental health issues are obvious, Lucas can be engaging with a wide, friendly smile. But first appearances are deceptive and belie the serious issues under the surface. Because of his good first impression, most people are fooled into thinking Lucas can be easily cared for and supported, even though they know his diagnoses. Since people have caring hearts; they are overly compassionate and giving. But these traits are exactly what Lucas uses to up his bad behavior. Because someone is kind and generous, he sees them as weak and easier to manipulate. The more we give, the more he expects and demands. And the charm fades.

CHAPTER 20

Making Friends with the Devil

Psychotic behavior is altogether different from ordinary bad behavior. This is when support really gets difficult.

I have worked in the field with mental health clients for over sixteen years and personally lived with schizophrenic clients for over nine years. There are different treatment therapies available, but these are supplementary. Medication is critical to manage the disease, but medication alone will not do the trick. My goal is not to delve into medications or therapies. My goal is to help you understand the nuts and bolts of this life changing disorder by giving a first-hand observer's view on the challenges one faces in living with someone who has this diagnosis.

When I first began working with clients with schizophrenia who had auditory hallucinations, I did a little research and observed psychiatrists as they worked with my people. I was surprised to discover that there were no definitive ways other than medication to handle the voices. I noticed that during psychiatric visits only one question was asked: do you see or hear things that may not be there?

The client would respond yes or no, and that was the end of the conversation. The only treatment suggested was medication.

Since I could find nothing to guide me, I decided I would fall back on what I knew best—observing and asking questions. I needed to know what was actually in Lucas's head before I could address it. I waited a few months until I felt I had built up trust. If I went in prematurely with probing questions, I expected to either get blank stares or be told it was none of my business. Patience paid off.

Lucas had "tells." He indicated by specific signs that he was headed toward a full-blown psychotic episode. He started with irritability and moodiness. He wanted to dress in black, and he talked about wanting a pale, white body and long hair. Sometimes his smile became "frozen." This could be interspersed with odd, almost hysterical laughter. He would pace with his head down, muttering and blocking out everything to concentrate on the voices.

When I saw Lucas muttering to himself or grinning without an obvious cause, I knew the voices were talking.

Sometimes he would respond to my questions at that point. But often it was more productive to catch him when he was in a good mood and there were no voices actively speaking in his head. We were driving in the car one afternoon and Lucas suddenly began laughingly uncontrollably in the back seat. I glanced in my rear-view mirror and saw him making odd motions with his right hand.

"Lucas, why are you laughing?" I asked.

Barely able to speak, he giggled out, "The leprechauns got pinched!"

I couldn't help myself; I had to ask.

"Who pinched them?"

"DR JEKYLL!" He dissolved into gales of laughter.

Another tell that often preceded psychosis was Lucas's grooming. He would have to take a second shower. He couldn't remember to use soap or brush his teeth. Or he would get out of the shower with dirty hair. His mind was distracted by voices.

Most of the time, Lucas got serious when the voices came into his head. He tried to block out everything else around him. If I interrupted the conversation he got angry. He often began by shouting, "Leave me alone!" Then he started cursing.

In our house, we have been called every name you can imagine. Douche bag, snot face, fat, ugly, and many more that I will not repeat. If these didn't get a reaction, then he escalated his language. It became more vulgar with obscene gestures for emphasis. Then the threats would start. He would threaten to "do something bad to you after you go to sleep." He had threats that he used repeatedly.

"I'm going to break your cell phone," he would yell, as he lunged forward, trying to grab it out of my hand.

"I'm going to get two bodyguards to take care of you."

"I will burn it [the house] all up," he yelled, as he shook his fist in my face.

At this point, he started throwing things around, breaking things. He knocked books off shelves and tried to pull the bookshelf over. He picked up whatever was nearby and chucked it at me. Even though he was psychotic, my job was to stay close and make sure he didn't hurt himself. He would throw trash all over his room and shove his television to the floor. I observed, however, that he never threw his superhero action figures. Not even once. They were his most prized possessions.

During particularly unstable phases, I had to remove the knobs from my gas stove and hide them when not in use. I also locked up knives and scissors. Psychotic behavior is unpredictable.

Eventually, I discovered that the voices had distinct personalities.

Most were male. I only recall one female voice, Barbara. She was bossy. Lucas was being silly while he cleaned his bathroom. She told him to stop it. He giggled and repeated after her, "Stop it, stop it, stop it."

Tom Cruise visited once. Lucas was in the upstairs hall, walking back and forth and laughing out loud. This was interspersed with muttering. I asked him why he was laughing. The laugh was not a happy laugh but sounded creepy.

"Hey Lucas, what's so funny?"

"Nothing," he said, and continued to laugh.

"But something must be funny," I said. "Tell me."

"We were thinking about something," he replied.

"Who is we?" I asked.

"Me and Tom Cruise. We think it would be funny to push you down the stairs and watch you go thump, thump, thump." He erupted into loud laughter.

I eased away from the top of the staircase, trying to put a little distance between us.

Then there was Lucifer. He had been Lucas's best friend since he was about five years old, according to his grandma. He could not, or would not, describe what Lucifer looked like in detail. Some of the voices had physical bodies that he described; others did not. For years he refused, but then one day he told me Lucifer had horns and a tail. He stopped suddenly, realizing he had told me something Lucifer didn't want me to know.

Lucas had a love/hate relationship with religion. He had a favorite preacher and liked going to church. He liked to hear the Bible stories and got irritated when he was not stable enough to attend. But one Sunday after lunch, he got upset about something, stood in the kitchen, and looked up toward the ceiling. He screamed and shook his fist at God. He said he was tired of being good, and from now on he was going to be evil. No, he was going to be an "abomination." His interactions with Lucifer were frequent at this time. He was either "into" religion or "into" the occult.

Lucas loved witchcraft. He loved spells and witches. He told me once that his dad was a warlock. Something as seemingly innocent as a Scooby-Doo cartoon would set off obsessive thoughts about witchcraft. He delighted in blood and gore and gravitated toward horror everything: movies, car crashes, graphic novels, vampires. He fixated on sharks and flesh-eating dinosaurs. The story of Zeus eating his five children made his eyes sparkle. He talked excitedly about Kurt Cobain's suicide. His favorite band was Nirvana. I was never a Nirvana fan, so I looked at some of their lyrics. Alarming word pictures. Songs like "Lithium," "Rape Me."

Lucas drew lots of violent, disturbing pictures. I have seen several where he drew himself killing someone, blood dripping from the knife. In others, he decapitated someone and held a bloody head in his hands. These explicit drawings became much worse during psychotic episodes. At times, they were drawings of people he knew, including me.

Lucas had a history of nightmares, or "visions," where "angels" came at night and talked to him. "Ha, ha Lucas, it's time to die." He wrote down disturbing thoughts such as, "I want to cut my mom's heart out and eat it."

One psychotic interaction with Lucifer involved a ritual. I heard unidentifiable, repetitive noises coming from his bedroom. I knocked, then opened the door.

His room was trashed, items slung everywhere. His closet doorknob was broken, and there were piles of clothes, shoes, and papers. Lucas was standing in the middle of his bed, dressed only in black pants. He had used a black Sharpie to draw a large pentagram on his bare chest. Some substance was smeared all over his arms and face. He had urinated in his bed and was jumping up and down, over and over, in the same spot. He was wild-eyed and continued to jump as I entered the room. The sounds I had heard were bed springs breaking. I watched for a moment, then spoke.

"What is going on?"

"I have to do this," he said, robotically. He kept jumping, staring at the wall in front of him. "They told us to do it," he continued.

"Told you to do what?" I asked.

"How to be evil and angry like Venom. How to *be* Venom." (Venom is a comic book character, an evil nemesis of Spiderman. Lucas fixates on Venom.)

"Who is 'they'?"

"Lucifer. Lucifer told me what to do."

"Who is 'us'? Who was he talking to?"

"Me and my voices."

"What did Lucifer tell you?'

"He said to clean myself. He said to put alcohol on my face and arms." Lucas was still jumping, up and down. In the same place.

"I couldn't find any," he continued, "so I used Clorox wipes."

"The ones we keep in the bathroom?"

"Yes." He spoke in a monotone voice; flat, unengaged.

"What did you do with the wipes?"

"I took off my clothes and washed my body."

"Okaaaaay. What is that other stuff on your skin?"

"Hair gel."

"Why?"

"Lucifer told me to purify myself."

“What else did he tell you?”

“To put on black clothes and practice clinching my fists.”

“Lucas, I am trying to understand. Why do you want to be evil like Venom?”

“Because I’m weak. Because I am not human.” He was still jumping on the bed, pausing occasionally to catch his breath.

“How did the bed get so wet?”

“I filled my trash can with water and dumped it out.”

“Why?”

“Because Lucifer told me to. He is my friend. No one else understands me.”

I noticed a second pentagram drawn on the back of his left hand.

“Ok, I think I understand. Let’s get off the bed now and get cleaned up.” It had been about fifteen minutes since I first heard the noise coming from his room. I had asked questions slowly and deliberately, sometimes waiting for his delayed answer. I wanted to deescalate the situation as well as get all the information I could.

“I don’t want to. It worked; I feel evil.” He continued.

``“I told them,” he said. “I told the spirits.”

“Who are the spirits?”

"Max," he replied."I told Max. Max said 'Lucas, I'm afraid of you.'" (According to what Lucas told me later, Max was either his half-brother or a foster brother.)

My brain reeled from this surreal conversation.

I approached the bed; Lucas was still jumping but now it was sporadic. I held out my hand, coaxing him to take it, and he stepped down to the floor. As I helped him get cleaned up, I noticed pee in the corner trash can.

I took Lucas to the ER for an evaluation, and he was transferred to a psych ward for a thirty-day stay. His medications were adjusted, he cycled back to his personal normal state, and he returned home. Whenever he became psychotic, this was the procedure we followed.

Living with a schizophrenic was a bit unnerving. I would make progress on one specific behavior, things would calm down, and then another unpleasantness would surface out of nowhere. It was sometimes next to impossible to determine if this was psychotic behavior or deliberate misbehavior, But most times it was as clear as a bell.

After a while, his support team decided Lucas was stable enough to go to a sheltered workshop. He had been asking for months. The workshop provided simple contract work for the clients. They sat at a common table in a small warehouse counting small items to put in plastic bags. The work was simple, and although the paycheck was small, Lucas loved going to the workshop. It was a chance to make new friends. We decided to start with three days a week. A van picked him up and off he went.

Within a few days he had met a girl he liked. I reminded him that he had to make appropriate conversation. We even practiced topics to talk about. I got specific. You can say she has on a pretty dress, but you may not comment on body parts. You can tell her you like her smile. You can ask her to be your friend. You may not discuss sex. This is a workshop, I kept reminding him.

Within two weeks, he had asked her to have sex with him. She went home and told her grandparents, who were understandably livid. We had more conversations about appropriate speech, but he ignored all the warnings. And sure enough, he was asked not to return. He was too much of a distraction.

When he was asked to leave the workshop, Lucas fell apart and blamed God. He said he wasn't going to be good anymore. He was going to be a "bad person." He began to express more interest in the occult, and his drawings became more violent, including one of me being hung by the neck with a rope. He would scream and curse with no immediate trigger. He started making racist comments toward my sons, cursing them with vulgar names. His property destruction increased, and he broke things in his room: a chest of drawers, a headboard for the bed, and a closet doorknob. He often had an odd "fixed" smile on his face.

Tonight, he talked to a new friend in his head. Lucas went to bed about 9:00 pm but didn't go to sleep. I heard him talking from the living room, but I couldn't understand what he was saying. As the minutes passed—fifteen, thirty, forty-five—his speech became more rapid and intense. Not a good sign.

"Lucas," I called out.

"What?" He came to his door and looked down over the loft railing to where I was working down below on my laptop.

"Why don't you come down," I said. "You seem to be having trouble sleeping. Who are you talking to?"

"My friend Drew."

"Well, come downstairs for a bit. Why don't you work on your puzzle?"

"I don't want to."

"I know, but you need a distraction to relax you so you can sleep. We have to get up early tomorrow."

He walked downstairs, glaring at me as he headed toward the kitchen table. He sat down in a chair with the puzzle in front of him. He sat still for maybe five seconds before he erupted, banging on the table.

"I AM HUNGRY. I AM HUNGRY. I AM HUNGRY."

"Okay. Please stop yelling."

"I AM HUNGRY. "

His expression suddenly changed; he jumped up from his chair and ran through the house, down the front steps, and out the door. He almost ran into a delivery guy from the pharmacy who was approaching the door with newly prescribed medication. The man looked stunned as Lucas rushed by, out into the street.

"I am assuming," he said, "that I'm in the right place."

"Yes," I said, nodding my head, as we both watched Lucas run down the street in the darkness.

A young female police officer soon found Lucas and brought him home. She got him out of the car. He stood there in his sock feet, sweatpants, and Marvel t-shirt.

"Let's go inside," she said to him. "It's cold out here."

"NO," he replied loudly. He glared at me.

"I don't want to live with her!"

"Let's go inside and talk about it," she said.

She took his arm. He started resisting her, and I took his other arm. He twisted and pushed against me, clawing at my hands, jabbing with his elbows, bending my fingers back.

A second officer arrived. This one was male, maybe forty, and tall. Releasing my hold, I stepped back, and he took Lucas's arm. They asked him what was wrong, why he ran.

"I was talking to my friend [voice]," he said, "and I don't want to live with *her*." He talked to the officer, but he didn't take his eyes off my face.

"I HATE HER."

Two police cars, two officers, Lucas, and I were in the street in front of my house for the second time in five days. Wonder what the neighbors thought.

He pulled against them, but they got him in the front door and up the few steps to the living room. He quickly turned, grabbed a large painting off the wall, and tossed it down the stairs. They grabbed him again. The male officer was firm but kind.

"Lucas, look at me. Look me in the face."

Lucas turned to look at him.

"You are a man," he said. "A man. What you just did is what a boy does, not a man. Tell me you won't do that again."

Lucas mumbled under his breath.

"Tell me," the officer repeated.

Lucas spoke quietly. "I won't do that again."

"Good," the officer said, relaxing his grip.

Immediately, Lucas lunged forward and grabbed a large sofa cushion. He threw it hard at the coffee table scattering my grandson's Lego creation everywhere. I eased over to a nearby desk and quickly removed my laptop and a large vase of flowers.

. The officers, grabbing both of Lucas's arms, sat him at the kitchen table in front of his Mario puzzle, one on each side of him.

"I like your puzzle," one of them said. "Tell me about it. "

Lucas just sat there.

"This is a nice house," one of them said. "A great place to live."

"I DON'T WANT TO LIVE WITH HER."

"Where do you want to live?"

"There is no place," he said. This time he didn't yell.

Lucas suddenly stood up, reached across the table, and knocked off his medication box. Pills flew across the room. I had been checking Lucas's medication when he ran off.

The officers grabbed his arms again while I cleaned up the mess. We all looked at each other, trying to figure out the next step.

"What do you want us to do?" the male officer asked.

"You will have to take him with you," I said, "there is no way I can control him when you leave."

EMTs came and took him to the emergency room first and from there back to a psych ward.

Lucas's grandma said she was afraid of him sometimes. I could tell she felt bad about that, but there was something to be afraid of. He once held a knife to his mom's throat and attacked her multiple times.

Lucas can, to some extent, minimize the voices in his head. What I have observed is that sometimes when the auditory hallucinations surfaced, he got angry and wanted them gone. I encouraged him to try to ignore them and fill his mind with other things like books, video games, puzzles. When he was proactive and told them to go away, they receded and might disappear completely *for a time.* The biggest problem was when Lucas didn't want the voices to go away.

For instance, when he was hospitalized for a med change and stayed several weeks for stabilization, his lack of distractions and normal life experiences allowed him to develop deeper friendships with the voices. He didn't want to give them up, although eventually the medication would win. Normally, he didn't mind taking his meds, but when he wanted to keep his voices, he would get agitated and question repeatedly what they were for. We were careful to speak generically and not tell him they would help his voices go away because then he might refuse to take them. Other times, he wanted all of them to go away except Lucifer. Never Lucifer. He called Lucifer his "best friend."

CHAPTER 21

Stepping out of Reality

Lucas collected coloring books, DVDs, books, and anything else that had superhero characters, especially bad ones. He liked to mimic them. On one occasion, he painted his face white and green with a marker so he would look like the Joker, because he wanted to be evil too. The look he was going for was the Heath Ledger look with the diabolical, sinister half-smile, not the old-time Joker my kids grew up with. Lucas dressed in black jeans and black t-shirt before he applied the markers to his face. He equated black with evil, with darkness. If he decided to be a villain after something didn't go quite the way he wanted, he would change his clothing to all black—so I removed it. It made him angry. And Lucifer too, I expect.

Another character Lucas loved was the Hulk because he "gets angry and loses control." Lucas had an uncanny knowledge of all the Marvel characters, even the more obscure ones and all their superpowers.

He loved Venom, one of Spiderman's enemies, and he grinned gleefully when Venom did something especially evil. Sometimes this was just childish mimicry; at other times it was the result of a psychotic episode. We had to block all access to Superhero movies, video games, and any related paraphernalia.

"What about the old Batman and Robin series?" I once asked his psychiatrist. "You know, the one with "POW" and "BAM" in bubbles over their heads?"

"Not even those," he told me. Lucas put on the evil characters as easily as the Pokémon pajama pants he put on before bed.

When Lucas wanted to step out of reality, my presence got in the way. He wanted to be alone. He paced back and forth. If I directed him outside to walk off anxiety, he would pace along the fence, over and over. He wore the grass away as he walked briskly with lowered head, running his right hand along the length of the wrought iron fence. He paced until he was tired, sometimes for as long as two hours. He didn't normally have a good sense of time but when he was psychotic, he lost all track of the hours passing. The conversations between him and the people in his head kept him occupied. If I tried to redirect his attention or otherwise break the spell they had over him, he got angry.

"LEAVE ME ALONE!" Lucas would shout. "GO AWAY. LEAVE ME ALONE!!"

He got belligerent over little things; he lost patience. He glared at me defiantly. He wanted to pick a fight.

"NO," he said, firmly, "I don't want to take a shower this morning."

"Yes," I replied, "you need to take a shower before breakfast."

"I won't," he said firmly as he glared at me. I tried to reason with him.

"Well," I said, "we both have our jobs. Your job is to take a shower. My job is to make you breakfast."

"What do you mean?"

"Your job is to take a shower," I repeated. "My job is to make breakfast. If you don't do your job, why should I do mine?"

"I hate you," he said.

"Just get a shower," I replied.

He stalked off to the bathroom telling Tom Cruise, or whomever was in his head today, how mean I was. I headed to the kitchen to make breakfast.

Lucas had a strong dislike for other people with disabilities. He attended a monthly get together, a social and advocacy opportunity for people with intellectual disabilities. Like Lucas, many were dually diagnosed with an intellectual disability as well as a mental disorder.

"Try to make friends," I said as we walked in.

"OK," he replied.

In a room with about sixty peers, Lucas looked for those who were *not* like him—personal aides, food servers, state employees. He ignored peers who would love to spend time with him; he thought he was better than they were, that he was special. He once made fun of a man in a wheelchair who was leaning to the side, drooling from his needed medication. And he could be racist. He used this when he wanted to get under my skin.

"Your sons are n*****s."

I tried to ignore him. He wasn't having a psychotic episode. He wanted to show me he was bad, and this was dramatic theater.

I realized the extent of his dislike of people with disabilities when I took him to see his adoptive mom. Ellie was in a wheelchair, unable to walk or efficiently use her arms, barely able to speak after coming out of an eight-month coma. It was the result of a surgery gone wrong. She motioned for Lucas to follow her into her room. A few minutes later, she wheeled herself out, crying. She wanted to give him $20 but he got frustrated at not being able to understand her clearly, shoved her wheelchair out of the way, and stormed out. When she died a year later, he never shed a tear, never asked about her. I waited for weeks thinking I might see a delayed reaction of pain, or sorrow, or anger, anything. But it never came.

Reactive attachment disorder is what they call it. Some of the symptoms in adults include detachment, inability to show affection, withdrawal from connections, and inability to maintain significant relationships whether platonic or romantic.

Lucas used people. He did not bond with them. Even an offer of help would soon be followed by something he wanted. Sometimes he enjoyed being difficult. Rules applied to others, not him, and he had a strong sense of entitlement. He hated the word "consequences" and got mad when I used it.

"But I don't want consequences," he told me many, many times.

"It's a natural part of life." I said. "Both good and bad, depending on choices you make."

He went off to his room to sulk.

Lucas has a new voice today named Krum. He is fat and has a unibrow. They talked about a book

Lucas was reading, *Diary of a Wimpy Kid*—something about a shoe chasing them. He reads at about a fourth-grade level.

One of the challenges of dealing with someone like Lucas is figuring out what is just bad behavior and what is psychotic behavior. The first requires accountability and consequences; the second requires treatment. Brand new social workers often get taken advantage of by clients who are not having a mental health problem but just exhibiting poor behavior. I have seen police officers, medical doctors, and even a mental health judge whose compassion led them to actions that not only didn't help the individual involved but assured the acting out would continue in the future. Experienced mental health workers or caregivers can usually tell the difference.

It is often difficult to know what triggers a psychotic event. One time when Lucas visited his grandparents, he took off his clothes and sat naked in the front yard all afternoon, refusing to go inside or get dressed. Eventually, he put his pants on but not his shirt. He was difficult all day, and when it was time for him to be picked up to go home around dark, he headed into the woods near the house. Grandma tried to get him out, but as she entered the edge of the woods, he just went in deeper. She called me and I made the hour-long trip to assist.

By now it was totally dark, and he was still in the woods. We sat on the carport in lawn chairs watching the woods, waiting for Lucas to come out, but he didn't. Finally, after a couple of hours, I said we probably needed to call the sheriff. A little while later, two deputies showed up. We explained the situation. I noticed they didn't appear to be in a hurry and in fact seemed reticent to approach the woods at all.

"It's alright," I assured them. "He's a little guy, and he has no weapons. You're not in any danger. He's been acting up all day. Just go tell him to come out of the woods or you're coming in after him. I think he will just walk out when he sees who you are."

"Maybe we need to call the canine unit," the officer said.

I later found out that many years earlier, while Lucas was still living with his adoptive mom, a dog had to be used to locate him deep in another woods. In fact, the city named one of the canines after him. An old newspaper photo shows the officer and his dog that found Lucas. Next to them is Ellie, tightly holding Lucas against her to try to control him, probably to keep him from running off again.

"You won't need it," I said. "He's at the edge of the woods."

They walked over to the edge of the woods and shone their flashlights. I couldn't hear what they said, but a minute later, Lucas walked slowly out, and they led him up to the carport. He was sulking.

"Lucas," I said, "it's ten o'clock at night. Come over here and put your shirt on."

Slowly, he did, glaring all the while.

"Why did you go into the woods?"

No response.

“Tell me what’s going on.”

Still no response.

“OK then. You owe everyone an apology.”

Nothing.

I spoke firmly.

“Apologize now, please. These officers have left other responsibilities to come here and get you out of the woods.”

A reluctant “I’m sorry” came out of his mouth.

“Now apologize to your grandma. You had her worried sick.”

“I’m sorry,” his mouth said, but his face told another story.

“It’s ok, honey,” she replied.

“No, it’s not, it’s not ok. Please don’t tell him that,” I said.

One of the deputies spoke up.

“Son,” he said, “if you ever go into those woods again and make us come get you, you will spend a night in jail. You hear me?”

Lucas nodded, but the officers and I both knew that wouldn’t happen. They have protocols to follow in situations like these.

“Say ‘Yes Sir,’” I instructed. “These deputies have real business they need to attend to, and you took time away from their jobs. You need to show some respect.”

"Yes Sir," he mumbled, looking at the ground.

The officers left.

"Lucas, tell your grandma goodbye and get in the car. We are going home."

He opened the back door and got in. After an occasion when he angrily tried to grab the steering wheel while I was driving, he was relegated to the back seat. The child locks were engaged because once he opened the car door and threatened to jump out while we were going seventy mph. When we got back on the interstate, I asked him what was wrong.

No answer.

"Why did you take off your shirt?"

"Lucifer said if I want power, I have to take my shirt off."

"What kind of power?"

"Like Venom."

We rode in silence for a few minutes. In the back seat I heard loud muttering.

"Lucas, what are you saying?"

"SHUT UP!"

"Who are you talking to?"

"Shut up, shut up, shut up."

"Lucas, don't talk to the voices. Talk to me."

"NO. LEAVE ME ALONE."

I saw him in the rear view mirror. His face was contorted with anger. I knew it was directed at me. "Who are you talking to? Is it Lucifer?"

"SHUT UP! I can't hear what he's saying when you talk."

I shut up.

As soon as we arrived home, I gave him his medication and he went to bed, still angry, but he slept through the night.

Police officers are wary of those with obvious mental health issues. They don't understand them, and what they/we don't understand, they/we fear. I was driving, before the steering wheel incident, on the highway. Lucas was beside me, sitting in the passenger seat of the car. He was quiet, hands placed palm down on each knee, staring straight ahead at nothing, mouth gaping open. Open road, no traffic. My mind wandered and my foot got heavier on the gas pedal. A blue light appeared behind me, and I slowly pulled over, my mind coming back to reality. Oh no. I suddenly remembered I had not yet renewed my car registration.

The officer approached my window and I spoke first. "I am so sorry," I said.

He glanced over at Lucas, still staring straight ahead, mouth gaped open, lost in his head. Rigid. He took a step back.

"I'm so sorry," I said again. "I know my registration is expired."

He bent down and looked in the window, past me to Lucas, who still hadn't moved. He took another step back, looking rather uncomfortable.

"Do you want to see my driver's license?" I asked, moving to pick up my purse.

No, he didn't.

"Ma'am, I stopped you because you were doing 80 mph in a 60 mph zone."

"I truly am sorry," I said. "I didn't realize how fast I was going."

"Where are you going in such a hurry?" he wanted to know.

He wasn't looking at me even though the words were meant for me. He was still watching Lucas. I nodded toward the passenger seat.

"I'm taking him to see his behavior analyst," I replied. The officer took a third step back away from the car.

"I'll get my license for you," I told him.

"No. No, that's OK. Just slow down and take it easy, OK?"

By now the officer had backed up even further and turned quickly, walking to his car. He drove off. I sat there for a moment. Expired registration and twenty miles over the speed limit. And he didn't even ask to see my license. Why? As I glanced over at the passenger seat the answer came to me. Lucas. The officer was afraid of Lucas, all of 5' 8" and 155 pounds of him. I guess he considered him unpredictable. Which, of course, he was.

A daily problem we had to address was that Lucas had no cut-off valve when it came to food. He would eat until he threw up. For two years I thought he was allergic to chocolate because it was documented as part of his medical history. Eventually, I discovered he had binged on chocolate until it made him sick, and someone mistook that for an allergy. It was entered in his notes, made it on to official documents, and would probably take an act of Congress to remove.

Lucas stole food. He would eat a large dinner, and a short while later sneak food, eat it, and then flush the wrappers down the toilet. Major plumbing issues and flooding always found him out. He would take food out of the trash can. He got choked on a Cheeto one time that he found in the garbage, and I had to dislodge it from his throat. He fought me while I was attempting to help him; even after he spit it out he was angry because he had been caught eating out of the trash. He tried to fight me, and my adult son had to step in. He didn't even think about the fact that he was choking and needed help. He kept saying I had mistreated him.

Lucas remembered past events by marking them with food. Last birthday? Logan's Roadhouse. Two weeks ago, Sunday? Steak and Shake after church. Peer get-together? Slice of pizza, chips, and chocolate chip cookies. Visit to Grandma's? Doritos and soda. My mother's house in Alabama? Ryan's steakhouse, pecans, and blueberries. Lucas told me that when his mom adopted him, she took him to Waffle House. He said he ordered pigs in a blanket. When the order was brought out, he asked where the faces were. She told him "They have no faces." The pigs, that is.

"That was really funny," he told me.

He couldn't remember his own address, but he remembered where every item was located in the grocery store after only a couple of visits. He noticed the items on the top shelf that I rarely pay attention to. He asked for different things.

"Can we buy caviar?"

"I want crab claws for dinner."

"Miss Belinda, I like lobster."

He knew the high-price specialty items. That's what he wanted to buy.

"How do you know about all these expensive foods?" I asked.

"My mom used to buy them for me," he explained.

I don't know if that's true. Maybe. But then, maybe he saw the item on TV and was trying to manipulate me.

As mentioned previously, Lucas was drawn to horror. He had an unhealthy obsession with evil characters. In Sunday School, he paid rapt attention to the story of Adam and Eve in the garden. How wonderful, said a church lady to whom Lucas was relaying the story. "He loves the story of Adam and Eve," she said, approvingly.

I gave a faint smile, knowing it was not Adam and Eve that he liked to hear about, it was the evil serpent, Satan. And when he talked about the story later, his eyes glistened as he recounted the wicked snake. Lucas made inappropriate comments to women or girls if left unsupervised. I decided to see how he would do in a Sunday School class he wanted to attend. It was a small high school class that my teenage son attended, and the participants were all sitting in a circle. Lucas sat down, scoped out the girls, and turned to the boy next to him.

"Wow, these girls are pretty," he said loudly and without embarrassment.

"But their skirts are not short enough," he complained. "You can't see anything."

He didn't get to go back.

In some areas, Lucas improved quickly after he moved in with my family. But we had a much harder time with table manners; he wanted to eat with his hands. When I insisted on a fork, he would take his other hand and scoop food to pile on top of the fork. So, I taught him to sit on his left hand and eat with his right. The problem wasn't lack of skill but the fact that he couldn't stuff the food down fast enough. After a couple of weeks, he learned to keep his left hand in his lap unless needed to tear off a piece of French bread or eat a chicken leg. He learned to wipe his hands on his napkin.

With self-control lacking when it came to food, parameters had to be put in place. Ask for a snack, do not raid the pantry. Do not eat anyone else's food. If they leave it on the cabinet for a while, it is still their food. Do not eat out of the trash can. If you just had dinner, don't ask for a snack. If you just had breakfast, don't ask for a snack. If you just had lunch, don't ask for a snack. Don't talk about food all day. Talk about other things.

The first time I took Lucas to a Chinese buffet with the family, I learned the extent of his food obsession. Thinking we might have a problem since the food was unlimited, I decided to talk to Lucas in the car before we went inside.

"So, here's the deal. They have great food here. But we need to be reasonable and not greedy. You may have two plates of food from the buffet, plus a salad and dessert. One refill on your drink."

"But why can't I have more?"

"Lucas, I just described a lot of food."

"But I want more."

"That's greedy."

"But I want to get whatever I want."

"Think about this. You have two choices. Agree not to pitch a fit and eat what I suggested, or we will go home."

"You can't do that. Everyone else is already inside."

"Oh yes, I can. We can sit in the car, wait until they have finished eating, and then go home and eat a peanut butter and honey sandwich."

"You are mistreating me!"

I said nothing.

"I want to go eat."

He tried to open the car door, but the child locks were engaged. He yelled for a minute and hit the back of my seat. I started the car.

"What are you doing?"

"Leaving the restaurant."

"But what about the others?"

"I'll come back and get them later."

"ALL RIGHT, ALL RIGHT I will only eat two plates."

"Thank you. Now pull yourself together and calm down so we can go inside."

Five minutes later found us walking through the buffet line. Lucas, at least for this visit, accepted a reasonable boundary. But although this battle was won, the war was only beginning.

I have never known Lucas to turn down food, even if he has just eaten a huge meal. He will not only eat anything offered to him, but he will beg for more. He may have gone hungry at times when he was very young, although I can't verify that. But I do know that since he was adopted at age five, he has always been fed very well. In fact, one of the problems has been that family, care staff, and professionals have used food through the years as a way of controlling his behavior. Is Lucas irritable? Give him food. Is he threatening to hurt someone? Distract him by taking him to McDonald's. And buy him a twenty-piece chicken nugget meal with large fries, milkshake, soda, and apple pie. That will put him in a better mood. Is he belligerent because he has to take a bath? Take him to the nearby convenience store and buy him soda, beef jerky, and a moon pie. Even mental health professionals on psych wards often controlled his behavior with food.

When Lucas moved in with me, he weighed 242 pounds. When I took him to his new doctor for the first time, he told me to get the weight off. Stop the fast food, increase the exercise, and no sodas. Lots of water. We did what he said, except for fast food about once a week, and the weight just fell off, down to about 160 pounds. I didn't serve family-style but plated the food, and that, combined with eating a little slower, worked wonders. Lucas was proud of his new "skinny" body, but he didn't internalize any changes we made. After nine years, he will immediately revert to old habits unless he is closely supervised.

Lucas was also obsessed with certain celebrities. I knew little about his biological family before he was adopted, and since he told conflicting stories, I didn't know if Lucas himself remembered much about them. But through the years, Lucas fantasized about his "real" family. I have been told many times about his dad's identity:

"Duran, Duran is my dad."

"Ben Affleck is my real dad."

"My father is Andrew Garfield. My grandma told me this."

"Daredevil is my father."

"The English king says I have more than one dad and if one dies, I will have another one."

"My real dad is Wolverine."

And then there is this.

"My dad is dead by Mary. She killed him with a dagger. He raped my mom and begged and begged her not to kill him, but she killed him on the ground and with blood on her shirt, and he looked sad on the ground frowning." The alternate version of this story is that a woman named Julie killed him.

And he tells me about different mothers:

"Angelina Jolie is my real mom, and she lives in a castle."

"Courtney Love is my real mom."

"My real mom is Buffy the Vampire Slayer."

"My mom is named Julie Victoria and she is a cat."

Psychologists would probably have theories about Lucas's preoccupation with numerous celebrity family figures. I just know he has a rich fantasy life.

"Long John Silver is my great grandpa. He bought me McDonald's to eat in England. He gave me a Power Ranger watch and a Lunchable."

"The Punisher is my friend".

"Arnold Schwarzenegger is really Frankenstein."

"Harley Quinn has blond hair. She was at the psych ward with me."

It is difficult to tell whether Lucas actually believes what he says or if he is just pretending. But he will also tell you about himself.

"My real name is Peter Parker."

"I am really Ant Man."

"Lanny [former staff] found me in the river when I was a baby, and this was before I had a family."

"How I came to be famous is me meeting lots of women and knowing their mamas with my guy friends. Some of the girls tickle me with their two fingers, and the one girl Taylor was like a girlfriend to me. She rubbed my chest and stomach. My girlfriend Taylor, I saw her in a computer, smoking."

"I want to be a famous singer." (When I said I didn't know he liked to sing, he replied "I don't.")

Lucas couldn't be unsupervised around animals. He got a creepy thrill out of hurting them. Sometimes, he seemed to enjoy their company, and I would let my guard down. He would stroke the cat, and then when he thought no one was looking, he would press her down hard on the floor or the sidewalk. She would meow loudly and try to get away, and he would push down harder, grinning gleefully. I once saw him beat a small snake to death. I admit no fondness for snakes, but when I saw him continue to pulverize that snake into an unrecognizable pile after it was clearly dead, laughing all the while, it startled me to realize how much he enjoyed the violence.

The maddest I ever got at Lucas was when I saw him mistreat our dog. Governor was a one-year-old, sixty-five lb. golden lab that belonged to my adult son who lived with me. He was an inside/outside dog and needed space to run. He was hyperactive for his breed, and the back yard was large and fenced.

Lucas had had a difficult morning; he was uncooperative and irritable. I suggested he go outside and walk around the back yard to work off some of his frustration. He stomped out the door. I started to the kitchen and decided I needed to keep an eye on him due to his mood. As I walked out on the deck, I was horrified to see Lucas attack the dog. He picked up a large stick about two-and-a-half inches in diameter and struck Governor hard enough to knock him over on his side. He lay there, still, and then struggled to get up. I yelled at Lucas to stop.

Lucas looked defiant as I ran down the deck steps and grabbed the stick away from him. I was livid. This sweet, friendly dog loved people and his tail never stopped wagging. If Lucas had hit him about six inches higher up, he would have been dead: the blow would have landed on the side of his neck and broken it.

"What are you doing?" I raised my voice out of anger and fear of what might have happened.

"Nothing," he grumbled.

"Why did you hit the dog?"

"I didn't." Now he was getting belligerent and glared at me angrily.

"I SAW YOU," I yelled.

After I realized Governor was alright, just shaken up, I took Lucas into the house. "No more," I said firmly. "Pets are off limits from now on. Don't touch them, don't pet them, stay away from them."

"But why?" he asked, challenging me.

"Because you are mean to them," I said. "And you know there are always consequences for bad behavior."

"I HATE CONSEQUENCES."

I remembered a young woman whom I had on a caseload years earlier. She was also cruel to animals. Cruelty to animals and children is especially heinous, and in an adult indicates a total lack of empathy. It is a trait that can never be ignored. PETA believes that only sociopaths intentionally hurt animals. Maybe they're right, I don't know. But anyone who gets joy out of hurting innocent animals is sick. Just sick.

CHAPTER 22

Manipulation

To some extent, we all manipulate, or try to manipulate, both our circumstances and the people around us. It is a way by which we attempt to control our environment—or to put it more plainly, to get what we want when we want it. A narcissist excels at using manipulation to obtain power and exercise control. Those who are intellectually challenged with mental health issues are no different than the rest of us. But to the inexperienced person it can be unexpected and often overlooked.

Please remember that those within my experience are mostly adults. But whether they are eighteen or sixty-five, the ability to manipulate never ceases to amaze me. It can be simple or complex manipulation. Take Jason, for example.

Jason, age thirty-four, got a new video game. Jason *loves* video games. He has simple chores, and he gets regular encouragement to "do something productive today." He is unable to hold down a job due to various immature behaviors, so staff try to fill his time with some chores, volunteer work, socialization, physical activity, and fun things. He prefers to do only fun things; specifically, playing video games for up to ten hours at a time.

So staff wakes Jason up, and when breakfast is eaten and hygiene completed, the productive day begins. After dinner, Jason has free time until bedtime. He can play video games, work on hobbies, read, listen to music, whatever he chooses. But Jason doesn't want to be productive; he wants to play video games all day. He knows the direct approach to staff will not work. So he says this instead: "Hey, Miss Belinda, let's don't go out today. You look tired. You need your beauty sleep. Every woman needs her beauty sleep."

The unspoken thought is that if you are resting, I can do whatever I want, and I want to play video games all day. That is an example of simple manipulation. It is usually easy to spot and rarely works. But Jason tries.

Another example of simple manipulation is one that is used so often in our disability world that it can be considered a classic:

"Miss Belinda."

"Yes?"

"Can I call you Mama? I want to call you Mama."

Awwww. How sweet. Tugs on your heartstrings.

But you are not his mama. And you will soon discover that he has multiple mamas. In fact, any female he answers to he wants to call Mama. He has a biological mama, and often multiple foster mamas, and sometimes a step-mama. It is a way to endear him to you so he can get what he wants. "Mama, can I . . .?" And it is often done in public places.

A less common manipulative tool is faking seizures. This can be to get attention, to avoid a chore, or to get sympathy. A seasoned caregiver can recognize a fake seizure immediately, but if the attempt occurs out in public, there is usually someone around to rush in with sympathy and attention. I remember Bryan getting bored in church one Sunday morning. The preacher had only preached about 30 minutes but in his opinion, that was way too long. He was sitting next to me, and suddenly leaned over to speak in my ear.

"Miss Belinda."

I turned to face him.

"Shhh." I placed my finger on my lips.

"Whisper softly."

He didn't drop his voice at all.

"Miss Belinda," he said more urgently.

"What, Bryan?" I whispered back.

"I'm having a seizure."

Everyone around us could now hear this conversation.

"Bryan, you are not having a seizure," I replied, still speaking softly.

He got indignant and louder.

"I am too."

"No, you're not. You're fine and church is almost over. Shhhhh."

He stiffened his spine, sat straight up, and glared at me.

"I need to go out. I am having a seizure!"

By now, he had started to disturb those around us, and I knew I had no choice but to take him to the foyer. As soon as we left the auditorium, he headed for the water fountain.

"What are you doing?"

"I just had a seizure, so I need a drink of water."

"Bryan, if you can talk and walk, you are not having a seizure."

"But I did!!!"

"Well then, we need to go home."

"But you told me we are going to the Chinese buffet after church!" He was glaring at me now. He loved eating out on Sundays and looked forward to it all week.

"Well," I said, "that was the plan. But since you had a seizure, we need to go home and let you rest."

He pouted on the twenty-minute-drive home. But he never faked another seizure when I was around.

Stan fakes seizures too. He's not quite as obvious; he won't *tell* you he is having a seizure; he will lie down and refuse to open his eyes. You can call his name and shake him, but he will not move. He simply plays dead. I have seen him do this in a bed at the hospital ER when they were ready to discharge him and he didn't want to leave. The nurse couldn't get him up. She verbally told him to get up, and then gently shook him but he wouldn't move. She didn't know what to do. He was like a dead man. A two hundred-forty-pound dead man.

I walked over to the bed, pulled on his legs, and moved him sideways across the bed until his legs touched the floor. I shook him firmly and told him it was time to go. He ignored me until I said I was leaving, and he would have to walk the fifteen miles back home. Suddenly, he came up out of his "seizure" and got out of the bed. But to continue the act, he wouldn't open his eyes and groggily stumbled across the room and into the door. Deliberately. I know of another time an ER doctor slapped his face, hard, to make him open his eyes after nursing staff had tried for some time and failed to get him on his feet and out the door.

Jasper was a master faker when it came to seizures. He had never had a real seizure, but he had seen those who did, so he hammed it up when he wanted something and couldn't get it any other way. One day he wanted soda. Not a drink of water. Soda. I heard him hollering from his room.

"Miss Belindaaaa—I having a seizure!!"

Knowing that if he was talking there was no seizure occurring, I got up from my computer to go see what he wanted.

When I walked into the room he was sitting in his chair, a tall lanky thirty-something-year old. He had his head thrown back, tilted to the side, and his tongue was hanging out of the side of his mouth. His head was slightly shaking. He was *good.*

I called his name. "Jasper." No response. A little louder. "Jasper." Still no response. I took my hand and slapped him lightly on his cheeks, first the right then the left, and called his name again, a little more insistently. "Jasper!"

He jerked upright. "Stop hitting me," he yelled. "I want soda!!"

I am still surprised at the cognitive ability that a person with a measurable IQ of 47 can conjure up to manipulate someone into getting what they want. The mind is an amazing thing.

Sharie Stines, a California-based therapist, says that manipulative behavior involves three factors: fear, obligation, and guilt. Manipulating can be an attempt to bully you, or to make themselves appear the victim. "Manipulation is an emotionally unhealthy, psychological strategy used by people who are incapable of asking for what they want and need in a direct way. People who are trying to manipulate others are trying to control others."

I agree, except for one word in that sentence. Incapable. Most of my clients through the years have been fully capable of asking for what they needed or wanted. Manipulation was a tool used deliberately by which they believed their chances of getting what they wanted were increased.

In our world, lies told by those we try to serve is a huge problem. It gets in the way of us being able to provide appropriate care, and it is so common it often goes uncommented on. I refer to it as "The Pinocchio Syndrome." I believe it is the single most common manipulative tool we encounter among those whose intellectual disability is classified as moderate or mild. And it may well be the most common manipulative tool used by anyone, disability or no disability.

The only exception to using lying as manipulation that I have personally experienced has been with some with autism. For some reason, many don't seem to be able to lie. They are sometimes manipulative in other ways, but they seem unable to tell a direct lie. My grandson has Asperger's, a high functioning form of autism. He is fourteen and in all his fourteen years he has never been able to lie. He may avoid a question, refuse to answer, or simply say, "I can't answer that." One trait often associated with autism is seeing the world and everything in it, including speech, as quite literal. They have trouble with axioms, slang vocabulary, and metaphors. Perhaps this affects their ability to lie. I wonder. But generally, among those with developmental disabilities as well as severe behavior issues, lying is common.

Some lying can just be ignored. You can't call out someone who lies sixty times a day. But for some of my people, ignoring their lying simply doesn't work. It is not enough for them to lie and be ignored. They want validation. They will keep lying and insisting they are telling the truth. Their purpose is to get you to *agree* they are telling the truth. They want to know you believe the lie. They want to know they have succeeded.

Casey comes to mind. Casey lied more than he told the truth. It didn't matter what the subject was. He would lie to get out of trouble, lie to make someone else look bad, lie to get attention. He would lie so often in a day that I could believe nothing he told me. He would lie about what he ate and where he went, whom he saw. He would lie about health problems. He would lie about whether he had taken a shower. Once, when he ran off to an ER, he told the doctor he was anxious and upset because his fiancé had died. (He had no fiancé, and no one had died). But Casey fooled a lot of people with his lying, and this intermittent reinforcement outweighed the consequences of when he was caught. He would lie about interactions and relationships with people. He would lie to police and health officials. He would lie about lying.

Another manipulative tool that Casey used was speed, or rather lack of it. He moved like a sloth. A simple fifteen-minute outside chore would turn into three hours. Then, of course, he would complain about how long and difficult the chore was. At age thirty-two, he deliberately moved like an old man. And if he walked across the street and saw a car approaching, he slowed down his slow walk even more. It was as if he was daring them to hit him. Casey used this method to control others. Whenever staff took him shopping at Walmart, he would s-l-o-w-l-y get out of the car and walk inside. Since he was to stay near staff for supervision purposes, staff would have to try to walk as slowly as he did, which didn't work, because Casey would just slow to a stop in the middle of the parking lot or aisle. Since I know the purpose of the slow movement, this manipulative tool is particularly irritating to me. I tend to move quickly and decisively, and I give credit to the caregivers who must deal with this multiple times a day.

Back to lying as manipulation: in the population I work with, this often takes the form of false allegations. These allegations can be against anyone, but usually they are against staff. I would guess that nearly every person who has spent a lot of time in direct care settings with high functioning individuals (with behavioral issues) has at least once in their career been the target of false accusations resulting in an abuse investigation by the state.

Casey once got mad at his live-in staff and told others he had been threatened by a gun. It never happened. The staff didn't even own a gun. But it took a month for the state investigators to reach a conclusion of "unsubstantiated" on the abuse claim Casey made. In the meantime, a temporary living arrangement had to be made for Casey, and his falsely accused staff received no paycheck for the duration of the investigation placement. Staff decided they would no longer provide a home for Casey. Living with his manipulation was just too problematic. It would only be a matter of time until he did the same thing again.

I learned quite early in my career not to take everything told me as gospel. Marcus was bad about calling to tell me he had no food in his house. He would sometimes embellish this statement by whispering quietly on the phone because he didn't want his caregiver to hear and get himself in trouble. The first time in my social work career that I heard the "no food" line, it upset me, and I got in my car and headed over to the house. But when I got there, I found plenty of food in both the pantry and the refrigerator. The only things lacking were chips, ice cream, and soda.

So, when Marcus called again complaining about no food, I asked him to go to the refrigerator, open the door and tell me what he saw. After I realized he had plenty of food in the fridge, I repeated the instruction for the pantry. Everything he needed was there except junk food. Since he is diabetic, some items are limited and not kept in the house. But to Marcus, no sweets (or chips) meant he had no food.

One client of mine had a more uncommon manipulative tool that he used. He had a dissociative disorder and from time to time would have a psychotic episode. But on this occasion, he decided that having to do chores like sweeping or cleaning his own bathroom was not fair, and he needed a break. In his world, getting a break from normal living meant going to the ER so they would send him to a psych ward. There he got to eat snacks and watch TV all day.

So, Bryan decided to fake psychosis. He sat down on the stairs, looking irritated. As I walked by, he began to growl. It was not mimicry, like a childish, animal growl, but a low, eerie, guttural growl. I tried to ignore it, but the sound continued. I knew Bryan well, and simply told him to stop growling. I was NOT taking him to the emergency room. He glared at me and growled one last time as I walked away. And then it was over.

CHAPTER 23

I See Needy People

Not everyone a social worker has the opportunity to help is a client. We notice needs all around us; not when we first begin to practice but over time. We become more aware and sensitized to people and their difficult situations. We can often see indicators of issues that most people wouldn't recognize. I can't explain it, but I have always marveled at the people who come into my life whom I wasn't looking for or expecting. Not clients assigned to me, but random people needing a little help here and there. Maybe groceries, or some counseling. Maybe someone to talk to who can understand and sympathize with their predicament. Sometimes they seek me out. I feel like I have a blinking neon sign on my back inviting strangers to open up to me.

Once I was in a Dollar General store and a woman got behind me in line. She tapped me on the shoulder. I turned around. She was holding a package of men's underwear in her hand.

"Can you help me?" she asked.

"I'll try," I said.

"Do you think these would fit my adult son?"

"Well, how large is he?"

"About medium size," she replied.

Since the package she was holding in her hand was marked "medium," I told her probably so.

She continued, nervously. "I know it is odd for me to be buying underwear for an adult son, but he has problems. Do you know anything about schizophrenia?"

Yep, I did. Turned out her son had just been diagnosed, and she needed assurance that if she made sure her son followed the psychiatrist's medication regimen, his disorder could be managed. A brief conversation after checking out the underwear and she went on her way a little less anxious. That was easy, on my part, anyway.

I don't remember how I met Sissy, but she needed help. She, her sixteen-year-old daughter, her young son, and her daughter's baby were staying at La Quinta. They were from out of town, visiting Nashville, and had run out of money. She told me Traveler's Aid had helped them but not enough.

"What do you need?" I asked.

"Well, we don't have anything to eat."

"That can be remedied quickly. I will be back in half an hour."

I found a grocery store nearby and bought two or three bags of groceries, focusing on things that could be eaten cold or heated in the microwave she told me was in their room. When I returned with the bags, she left the room for a bit and I talked with her daughter, Mellie. Traveler's Aid had sent them to the women's rescue mission first, but her mom had been able to get donations from passersby so they could stay at La Quinta. This was their second day at the hotel. Suddenly, Mellie told me she thought her mom was going to drown her baby in the hotel swimming pool. After talking a bit longer, and asking some probing questions, I noticed signs of paranoia, so I wasn't sure how serious to take her fears. Her mom, Sissy, on the other hand, seemed strong willed and manipulative but not delusional.

When Sissy came back, Mellie stopped talking. The baby seemed healthy, and I turned my attention to the little boy. He was well fed, dressed in clean clothes, and his hair had been recently cut. Nothing unusual jumped out at me. His name was Ethan, but they called him "Little Man."

I gave Sissy my cell number and told her to call and let me know how they were doing. She called the next day.

"Ms. Mitchell," she said. "I need to take Mellie to the doctor. She was up all night throwing up. Can you bring me $40? I don't have enough money."

I sensed something was off but a few more questions got me nothing but more questions. "Ok," I told her. I took the money to her at the hotel.

The next morning, I called to check on Mellie. "How is she?" I asked.

"There's nothing wrong with her," Sissy replied breezily. "Guess what we did today?"

"Uh, what did you do?"

"We went to Madame Tussauds Wax Museum to see the country music stars. It was so much fun. I love Alan Jackson!"

I processed this in my head. Three tickets, not cheap, to the museum. I began to get irritated. At that time, money in my own family was tight and we were barely getting by. I had been tricked into paying for their museum tickets. I kept my cool because I wanted to find out more. I guess Sissy figured that she couldn't get anything else from me so she opened up.

Sissy's goal in life was to write a song that Alan Jackson would record. She wasn't really a songwriter, she told me, but she thought she could do it. "Alan Jackson is the best lookin' white man I've ever seen!" she gushed. (I thought that was an interesting comment since she and her family were also white.)

So . . . they came to town because of Alan Jackson.

(Insert heavy sigh right here)

We sometimes have an easier time opening up to strangers than to someone we know. I guess that is why through the years I have been approached so many times while standing in line at the grocery store. With no encouragement at all, words will spill out and soon I know much more than I ever wanted to know about the person standing in front or behind me. I have heard about the recent death of a friend or family member, or about a divorce or a cheating spouse. I have listened to sad tales of diseases and mental health problems. I have heard awful things, private things, spoken out loud simply because I was there and didn't turn away. There is safety in voicing anxieties to a stranger.

Make no mistake about it. If you help people, sometimes they will take advantage of you. And let's be clear here: not everyone deserves help. I spoke with a young couple about this just recently. They both are kind and compassionate. They want to do what they can to help others around them, especially those who have many more of life's challenges than they do at this stage of their lives. They had some of the same questions for me I have confronted myself.

How do I know if they deserve it? If I give money to a street person, will he/she spend it to feed their habit? How do I know if someone is lying to get a handout? What if they are not willing to work for it? What if they are in this country illegally?

Many people have these same questions. There is a basic instinct in most of us that makes us want to stand up for the underdog. Either we have experienced hard life struggles and feel at least some of their pain, or we feel a little guilty because our lives seem to be so much easier. But we don't spend our time or money lightly. So before we give, we want to know if they are deserving of our help.

Before I address this, I want to put a caveat up front: it depends on the situation. When I was in college and would ask my father hard questions, he often responded with, "it depends on the situation." It was not a satisfying answer, but now I see the wisdom in his response. He was not going to delineate a set of rules for me to follow. As I eventually came to understand, circumstances and relevant factors come into play. It depends on the situation.

That is my umbrella answer. Now I will give you my opinion on the above questions.

Question: How do I know if they deserve help?

Answer: You don't. You can't. And it doesn't matter.

I have never heard anyone struggling with an addiction, or living out of their car, or with a severe disability ask this question. Those of us with stable incomes, stable lives, and stable support are the ones concerned about it. Poor people know how it feels and will try to help each other. I spoke with a young man a few days ago who has been fighting an addiction and has lost everything, including his job. An old man asked him for money. He thought the man was lying and making up his story just to get a handout. But all the same, he pulled out all the cash he had and offered it to the man: a few dollars of change in a Ziploc sandwich bag. As he told me his story, I remembered a quote attributed to Johnny Cash: "Anyone who has suffered a lot of pain has a lot of compassion."

I do not deserve the blessings I have. I do not deserve my family, my health, or my home. I do not deserve a job I love or even the sun on my face. I do not deserve air conditioning in my car when the heat index, like today, is over 100 degrees. I do not deserve any abilities I was gifted with that have assisted me throughout my life. If I told you I did, you would consider me arrogant, and rightly so. Let's not be concerned about prequalifying people before we help them. They are not applying for a mortgage; they are asking for a little help.

Question: If I give money to a street person will he/she spend it on their habit?

Answer: Maybe.

Remember, there are only a few reasons people stay on the street for a long time. (There are also those with temporary situations that knock them down, but usually, social service agencies, churches, or extended family help get them back up.)

So if the person asking for help has been on the street for a long time and wants money, he may spend it on alcohol or drugs. But even people on alcohol and drugs need money to eat.

I would suggest that if you have any moral qualms about giving them money, give them something else instead. Maybe food. That's what I did in the beginning. But eventually, I decided that unless I knew *for a fact* the money was going to their substance of choice, I would just give them what I could and move on. And since I never had anyone in the middle of a drug deal or inside a liquor store approach me for money, I stopped worrying about it. I would never know. What I gave was a gift. I have always considered money with strings attached not a gift at all. It is a business arrangement.

For those of you who are still undecided, find another way to help. Be creative. In the summer I sometimes buy blankets from thrift stores. I wash them and put them away. When winter comes, I keep them in the trunk of my car and hand them out as needed. I used to keep a few umbrellas in my car to hand out when I saw someone standing on a corner in the rain. My kids have made personal hygiene bags to give out with small soaps, toothpaste and toothbrushes, shampoo, and baby wipes. Frozen water bottles in the summer are always welcome. If you don't feel comfortable with handing strangers money, figure out another way to help them. Do something to give hope whenever you have the opportunity.

Question: How do I know if someone is lying to get a handout?

Answer: You don't. Again, you do not have to prequalify them. This is not a loan. It is just a small gift.

Question: What if they are not willing to work for it?

Answer: Do you have work that needs to be done? An unskilled task that just anyone can do? Are you willing to provide transportation and supervision? Do you want to take the responsibility for someone you don't know who may have an unmanaged mental disorder or a substance addiction?

There have been times when I have offered work and was gladly taken up on the offer. There have also been a few times when I overestimated the ability of the person to complete the job, although they were eager to try. Mental disabilities are not always evident. I have seen couples with children who needed things, but although it was not readily apparent, both parents were unstable mentally and could not work.

The point is this: work situations in most cases are hard to navigate. If you know someone who is having a hard time and can work, offer them work. There is dignity and honor in honest labor. If you offer work, and they *look* able-bodied yet refuse, they may be lazy. But then again, they may have a mental disorder that is not obvious until you have been around them for a good while. At times, you may have someone ask you for help who *can* work but *won't.* People who are in dire need are just like the rest of us. Some are kind and grateful, and some are cranky or lazy. As a giver my job is to use wisdom and treat others the way I would like to be treated.

Question: What if they are in the country illegally?

Answer: I don't ask and don't care. That is their business, not mine.

I would love to be able to honestly say I have never broken a single law. But I can't. Have you ever:

Gone 70 mph in a 55-mph speed zone?

Picked up a hitchhiker on the interstate?

Taken your spouse's pills? (Both state and federal laws prohibit this)

Let your dog off the leash in a public place?

Failed to get your cat vaccinated one year?

Filed taxes late?

If we are honest, every single one of us breaks a law from time to time. We sometimes have a good reason, maybe even an excellent reason, so we feel okay about it. My point is this: unless you have never broken a single law, not even one, don't throw stones. We are all in the same boat. Maybe you broke a law due to an emergency. But that is also why many illegals cross the border. Their family is in a crisis, and they can't feed them. Or they fear for their safety.

When you are kind and take the time to develop relationships, immigrants will often open up and tell you their stories. Listen. *Then* decide if you feel comfortable passing judgment on them. And incidentally, crossing the border to seek asylum is not illegal. I know our immigration system is broken. I think it needs a complete overhaul. But I am not responsible for the immigration system; I am responsible for how I treat my fellow man. Compassion is always a good choice.

There is no substitute for one-on-one contact to understand another person's point of view. Too often we listen to politicians, friends, religious leaders, journalists, or family members to tell us how to act or what to do. We check out influencers or our favorite talk show host. We listen to everyone except the person with the problem who needs help. I hope it is not because deep down we don't want to get involved.

There are some needs that you will be unable to meet. Check resources in your community and refer people to someone who can. Speak kindly, and let people know you care. They won't forget.

CHAPTER 24

Volunteering

I was privileged for many years of my married life to be able to stay home with my five children and not have to depend on a job with wages. When I married my husband, we decided we wanted a large family, but I was the oldest of five and I knew what that would require. Caring for and training a lot of children was a full-time job. So, we made an agreement. He would work at his profession to provide our living, and I would care for the children and pretty much take care of everything else—household issues, filing taxes, paying bills, hiring repair techs, education, pet care, and everything else that comes with managing a home.

During the years when the children were young, we decided that since I was home anyway, we could take in foster kids. The urgent need at that time and place was for emergency care. That meant when there were no regular foster placements available, social services called us. Our home would be a temporary home until a more permanent foster placement became available. There were a few kids that I will never forget.

One of the first emergency placements was a girl, eleven years old going on twenty. Katie did not come from the typical situation; no drugs involved, no parents who had run afoul of the law. The issue was a failure to get along with her parents who had adopted her nine years previously. The confrontations between her and her mother started with disagreements over boys, makeup, and freedoms; common topics for mothers and daughters to navigate. But the arguments escalated, and things were smashed and broken. The social worker asked if I would let Katie stay with us for a while and see if I could figure out what was going on. Her parents were at their wits end. I agreed.

When the social worker brought Katie over, I noticed immediately she was very pretty, well-dressed, and friendly; a bit too friendly for her age and her new temporary living arrangement. She had uncommon poise for a child her age and came into our home as if she owned the place. Red flag. I got her settled and introduced her to my three young daughters. Katie liked to talk, especially about herself, so I was able to piece together a little of her story.

She was an only child. Her parents were quite a bit older than my husband and me, and she thought they were out of touch, not "cool." She also thought I was "pretty," and although she didn't say it out loud, I came to notice within a few days the attention she paid to my husband. Seems she thought he was "pretty" too. Another red flag.

It didn't take long to figure out that Katie liked to run things. She was given chores just like my daughters, and although she did them, I knew she chafed at responsibility. She always wanted to go shopping, go to the movies, do something fun. Although we went out several times a week, we also stayed home a lot. I wanted to observe her in a normal family structure. My brother, a college freshman, was living with us, so our household of seven was rarely boring.

I was in the kitchen cooking one evening, and the girls were entertaining themselves. My brother was watching TV, and it occurred to me I hadn't seen Katie in a little while, so I went to see what she was up to. I walked into the living room just in time to see her approach my brother and, without saying a word, sit down on his lap. He was startled and told her to get off. She continued to sit there trying to flirt as he kept telling her to move. I walked over quickly, and loudly and firmly told her to "get off of him." She slowly got up and sauntered away. She didn't seem the least bit embarrassed or remorseful. The red flags were beginning to accumulate.

Another time she stole my nine-year-old's eyeglasses, broke, and hid them. We all knew it was her, but she would never admit it. She lied about lots of things. In fact, because Katie seemed somewhat taken with my husband and brother, and was regularly deceitful about little things, we decided that we should take steps to protect our family in case she made some wild accusation. We knew by then what she was capable of and decided that neither man would ever be alone with her, even briefly.

She stayed with us a month. Although she knew the placement was temporary, she told neighbors we were adopting her. By now, I had figured out some things. First, the dynamic between her and her parents had to change. I was sure she had been playing her parents against each other, because she started doing that with my husband and me after only a week. It was a "divide and conquer" technique to get her way.

Next, her parents had to toughen up, especially her mother. They had to stop taking what Katie said so personally. Katie had been adopted at age three, so although she may have remembered her biological mother, I knew she didn't remember everything she talked about. She selected "stories" that were intended to hurt her adoptive mom. When Katie would get angry, she would tell her how much better her biological mom was and how she wished she could go back and live with her. The adoptive mom would fall apart; she would weep and wail, and sometimes throw things. Katie learned she was in control of the mood in her environment.

I picked up on this but not because of my education or training. It was personal experience. A few years earlier, my precocious four-year-old daughter tried the same thing. She was adopted at ten weeks and had never met her birth mother. She was an exceptionally bright, beautiful, lively child who, like every four year old, wanted her way, even when it wasn't good for her. I don't recall the reason, but she was mad. I had scolded her, and she wasn't going to let it go. This petite, little brown-eyed girl put her hands on her hips and glared up at me.

My birth mom was prettier than *you*," she said firmly, as she watched my face for my reaction. She was my first adopted child, and I wanted to be a perfect mother to her, with a perfect relationship. I was stunned. I just stood there, not knowing how to respond. She waited, lips pursed. After a few moments, I squatted down in front of her, so we were on the same level.

"I've never met your birth mom, Tabitha, but I think you're right. You are such a pretty girl; she *must* be beautiful."

She briefly looked puzzled, then smiled a little and ran off to play. She never tried that tactic again.

And being an insecure, young adoptive mom, I went to my room and cried.

There were other emergency foster placements, including a few infants. One sweet baby girl we only had for a few weeks. When she was born, the doctor suspected she had Down syndrome, and the grandparents who had planned to care for her didn't want a special needs baby. She came straight from the hospital to stay with us until the medical tests were run that ruled out Downs. Then her grandparents wanted her back. I only hope Claire never, ever found out that she wasn't wanted at birth because she wasn't "perfect."

I also remember a call late one evening after dinner.

"We have a six-month old we need to bring out right now," the worker said.

"What's going on?" I asked.

"There was an incident with his mother, and his grandparents don't want to take care of him," she replied. "And he's sick."

"OK. Bring him over."

Within thirty minutes, she showed up with a small bag and a blond-haired baby boy. He was screaming at the top of his lungs.

The social worker told me a little more. His mother had had a severe psychiatric incident while he was nearby. And by the way, the doctor said he has pneumonia.

"Pneumonia?" The baby was in my arms now, and still screaming. Screaming, not crying.

"Why wasn't he taken to the hospital?"

"The doctor thinks he will do better in a home setting. He's been traumatized."

I took a deep breath. My kids were already in bed, thankfully. This would be a long night.

As soon as she left, I began trying to calm him down. We walked the floor, I sang lullabies, tried a bottle. Maybe he's hungry. No, he's still screaming. Poor sweet baby.

We kept walking. Back and forth, back and forth; from one end of the house to the other we walked. Within about half an hour the screaming changed to soft crying. Finally, that stopped too. He was worn out. I decided to try rocking him to sleep. When I sat down in the rocking chair, I noticed something I had not focused on during all the screaming. He wouldn't bend his legs.

Mothers know that when you hold a baby on your hip, they fold their legs around your waist. Not Charlie. His legs were stiff as a board, hanging straight down as we walked. And when we sat down, only *I* sat down. He stood on my lap. I tried to cuddle him next to me. Nope. Those legs wouldn't bend. I stood up again and tried to cradle him against my hip. Nope. Still stiff-legged.

What was wrong with his legs? No one told me he had a physical disability. He looked fine. His legs were straight and well-developed. And when I sat down and he stood on my lap, there was plenty of strength in his legs. But I had to move on. He had pneumonia, and I had never cared for a child with that before. I pulled out my book on childhood diseases and looked up pneumonia. Not much advice beyond fluids and rest. Since he had stopped screaming, I could tell he was having some trouble breathing. It was irregular, and his little chest was caving in with each breath.

I remembered that in the past my mother had told me warm, moist air could help. I pulled out the vaporizer and filled it with water. With my husband's help, because I couldn't put Charlie down without him starting to scream again, we made a tent over the crib out of sheets, and soon the area around the crib was filling with the moist air. Now to get him to sleep.

It took another hour of walking and singing before I felt those little legs relax, cradling next to me, and a little head on my shoulder. So, there was nothing physically wrong with Charlie's legs. Whatever he saw or heard during his mom's psychiatric incident had terrified and paralyzed him. He was already in distress due to the pneumonia; then he was taken to a total stranger's house late at night. For an infant to be so traumatized hurt my heart. The rest of that night my husband and I took turns sitting next to the crib. There was no way I was leaving that baby alone. I was afraid he wouldn't make it through the night.

But he did, and the next morning his breathing was better. He stayed with us a few days until a more permanent foster home was found for him, and then he was gone.

After our two oldest daughters had gone off to college, I began volunteering once a week at a local soup kitchen. My family and I helped serve lunch to hundreds of homeless men each Tuesday. I worked on the serving line, dishing out whatever was donated for that meal. Both of my young sons worked nearby. The five-year-old handed each man a set of plastic flatware wrapped in a napkin while my eight-year- old poured drinks, usually water, into Styrofoam cups.

When we first started I was a little apprehensive about my sons volunteering with me, even though they were only a few feet away and always in my sight. But a man named Max allayed my fears.

He approached me shortly after we started working at the mission. He was a short, stocky man about forty, neatly dressed, and had been homeless for a long time before he got sober. He had succeeded in overcoming his demons.

Now he was there to help the others. And as he told me, he acted as bouncer whenever someone started getting out of line. I found out later he had been a pretty successful boxer in his younger years. That explained his look and speech pattern. It wouldn't have surprised me to find out he had some trauma from too many blows to the head.

"Miss Belinda," he began, "I know you might be worried about those boys of yours. I just wanted to say you rest your mind easy. I ain't gonna let nothin' happen to those boys."

"Thank you, Max." I didn't know what else to say. He continued.

"We don't put up with nothin' in here. If somebody starts something, I can handle 'em. They know I mean business. I'm good with my fists."

Knowing this both assured me and alarmed me. But he went on. I guess he thought I needed more convincing.

"This guy came in to eat a while back, and he was mouthin' off. I asked him polite like to settle down, but he thought he was tough. He got in my face, and I told him to back off 'cuz he didn't know who he was messin' with.

"Now Miss Belinda, I'm a Christian. I don't wanna fight no more. But he started cussin' and carryin' on. And people who come in here need protectin'. So I prayed, Lord, forgive me for what I'm about to do. Then I hit him. He was out cold and ain't been back since. So, your boys gonna be awright as long as I'm around."

We volunteered there for two years and nothing out of line ever happened to my sons. As I came to know a lot of the men, I realized there were many among them who would protect them if the need arose. And the boys were always within a few feet of me, never out of my sight.

My sons developed compassion toward those they served, especially the older one. One day while we were working the kitchen line, I looked over to see Andrew playing a little game with one of the homeless men waiting to eat. Andrew took three Styrofoam cups, turned them upside down, and placed a dollar bill from his pocket under one of the cups. Then he quickly moved them around and asked the next man in line to guess which cup the bill was under. The man looked over at me. He seemed uncomfortable. I smiled and told him to go ahead and guess. When he guessed the right cup, a big grin came over my son's face. He picked up the dollar bill and tried to hand it to the man.

"It's yours," he said. "Take it." The man shook his head. He wasn't going to take money from a child. But Andrew was insistent. After all, that was the point of the game: to give away his money to someone who needed it without causing embarrassment. "Go ahead," he said. "You won it fair and square."

The man hesitated, looking over at me again.

"Andrew is right," I said. "You won it fair and square. He wants you to have it."

He reluctantly took it from his hand and said thank you. Then he picked up his tray and moved on.

Many street people are at a soup kitchen or mission because they have an alcohol or drug addiction. Some, including many veterans, are suffering from post-traumatic stress disorder; alcohol and drugs are common ways to self-medicate the pain and anxiety. Others suffer from untreated mental health disorders. And homelessness makes no class distinction.

One of the men we served used to be in fiber optics. He was intelligent, articulate. One young man was the son of a well-known attorney; another wanted to be a country music singer. Many had physical problems, and one of the men had complications that led to his leg being amputated. Another had tried suicide three times but was still alive. The last time he had overdosed on his anti-depressant medication.

Mexican immigrants came through the food line occasionally, but rarely did we see them more than once or twice. They usually had just arrived in the US, or at least in Nashville, but had no money for food. They were waiting on that first paycheck. As one young man proudly told me when I offhandedly said I would see him next week, "No—you won't see me again. I have work. When I get my pay I buy my *own* food," he said in broken English.

And then there was Kenneth.

Kenneth probably had multiple mental disorders. I don't know what his diagnoses were, or if he had ever been professionally diagnosed, but he certainly had regular psychotic episodes. He had been on the street for a long time and always wore sunglasses. On Tuesdays when we showed up to serve lunch, Kenneth was often waiting outside the door. He would first speak to my sons and then address me. I never knew what to expect.

"I am Jesus Christ," he once loudly told me.

I just smiled slightly and said, "Hello, Kenneth."

"Jesus Christ," he repeated, waving his arms in the air. "I am Jesus Christ."

I knew better than to argue with someone who was clearly delusional.

"Well," I said. "It's about lunch time. You hungry?"

He nodded, and we went inside. But a few weeks later he was waiting for us again, and this time he was Bob Hope. Another time he was a witch doctor. Once he introduced himself to me as President Anwar Sadat of Nigeria. (Nigeria?) As I got to know him better, I asked if I could take his photo. With a head full of white hair, his brown skin, and dark sunglasses, he had a striking presence.

"No," he said, firmly. "You can't. My guardian angel has already taken my picture."

The conversations with Kenneth were, well, odd. When I first introduced myself to him, he repeated my name back to me.

"Your name is Belinda, not Lynda like in Lynda Carter who used to play Wonder Woman."

I started to reply, but he repeated himself.

"Your name is Belinda, not Lynda like in Lynda Carter who used to play Wonder Woman."

Again, I opened my mouth to speak. He continued to repeat the same sentence. Four times.

I got some friends to volunteer with me, and soon we all looked forward to interacting weekly with each other and the men we served. Sometimes we would sing in the serving line or tell jokes to the guys as they picked up their trays. Some of the men started looking for us and would make sure they came on the days we served lunch. They learned our schedules, and more than one of them told me they looked forward each week to us being there.

One day after we finished serving, I went into the dining area to start wiping tables. As I approached one table, I could hear a man telling a vulgar joke to the other men sitting around him. They were starting to chuckle. I decided to have a little fun, so I walked over, and leaned in toward the man.

"Ohhh." I dropped my voice to a loud whisper.

"Does your Mama know you talk like that?"

He looked at me, startled, and flushed. I smiled just a little, and walked toward the next table, dishrag in hand. As I started wiping it down, I became aware of someone coming up behind me and turned around. It was one of the men who had been listening to the dirty joke.

"I'm sorry, Miss Belinda," he said apologetically. "He's new. He don't know we don't talk like that on Tuesdays."

Perhaps the man who made the most impression on me was Liam. He was quite articulate and was usually found sitting on the floor or on the ground outside the mission with a sketch pad in his lap and colored pencils scattered all around. Liam sketched greeting cards, quite detailed and always with a poem. Many of his cards were religious in nature, and he included a Bible verse with each drawing. When he took a break from his sketching, he would sometimes pull a tattered Book of Psalms from his right pants pocket and read aloud to whoever wanted to listen. Psalms 148:1–14 was one of his favorites. It is a song of praise. In it, the psalmist is calling on the whole earth to praise the Lord; the sun, moon, and stars; mountains, hills, and beasts of the field.

Liam was homeless, had mental issues, and few possessions. He was different from most of the other men and stayed mostly by himself. He only wanted peace, and there isn't much for someone without a home. He was dependent on the kindness of strangers to buy his handmade greeting cards for his necessities, including the clothes on his back.

I took his photo as he sketched. Later, I made a print and took it to him. He was pleased and thanked me. "I've been told," he said, "that in my younger years I had a classical face. I suppose I still do." He smiled wryly, picked up his pencil, and returned to his work.

CHAPTER 25

Concrete Angel

Sometimes social services fail. That is why Penny was homeless from the time she was three years old until she turned twenty. She grew up on the streets in plain view of everyone passing by. Her mother exploited her, using her to panhandle. Through the years, dozens of calls were made to the local police department, who in turn called Children's Services. No one there acted on Penny's behalf. No one there investigated. The police department finally gave up, thinking there was nothing they could do. So she stayed on the streets. Occasionally, a cop would buy both mother and daughter a meal just to keep tabs on her.

The first time I saw Penny was in Panera. I was eating dinner with my brother and sister-in law when we looked up, and there she was. She had long, scraggly blondish hair and was dressed in baggy clothes several sizes too large. She looked about ten years old and was with an older woman I assumed was her mother. The woman, wearing layers of dirty, old, ill-fitting clothes looked to be in her sixties. She had a weather-worn face and appeared homeless. I looked closer at the girl. Almond-shaped eyes, compact body. She had Down syndrome.

They had come in through the side patio door and made their way over to the drink machine, where they filled their non-Panera cups. I noticed an employee watching them, but he said nothing. I guessed this was a regular occurrence.

After the pair refilled their drinks, they headed back toward the patio door. As they passed our table we said hello, and they stopped. We introduced ourselves. Penny's speech was difficult to understand, but her mother, Alice, said Penny was thirteen. Penny held out her small, grimy hand toward my brother and spoke.

"Cah," she said emphatically.

Penny folded her hands, placed them next to her face and tilted her head as if she was going to sleep. She pulled on my brother's sleeve and looked expectantly into his face. He looked quizzically at Alice.

My brother spoke. "I don't understand what she is saying."

"She wants a room key," Alice replied. "For a hotel room."

I realized she was referring to a plastic card, the kind that grants room access when you place it in the door slot.

One of us, I don't recall who, asked her if they had a place to stay that night. It was now fully dark outside. No, she didn't.

"Where do you usually stay?" I asked.

"Sometimes with friends," she mumbled.

"Do you have any money?" I inquired.

She hesitated, then uneasily said, "No," as she shoved her hands into her pockets.

"Are you sure?" my brother asked. I found out later he saw a large wad of bills inside a pocket of her skirt.

Alice looked straight at him, then looked away and nodded.

There was a hotel nearby, and we decided to get them a room for the night. We offered them a ride, but Alice said she had a car and would meet us there.

We drove over, and a few minutes later an old van pulled up. It looked like it was on its last leg. But what got my attention was the inside. It was filled to the brim with bags and bags of stuff. Alice was a full-blown hoarder, just like you see on TV. There was a small spot on the windshield left uncovered so the driver could see the road directly in front of her. The rest of the van, including the back seat, was filled all the way to the ceiling with junk. Penny had a small place to sit, but no way to see out either frontward or backward. She had to sit cross-legged; there wasn't even room for her small legs. I had never seen anything like it. It wasn't safe to drive.

They got out, and Penny started running around the parking lot. She was speaking, but with few words we could understand. She jumped around, ran back and forth, and laughed. I was unfamiliar with the hotel, and it occurred to me they might not want to give this homeless pair a room, especially since Penny was acting like a wild child.

I suggested that my sister-in-law go in with Alice and pay for the room while my brother, Penny, and I waited outside. After the transaction was completed, we would bring Penny in. Alice agreed.

While they were checking in at the front desk, Penny ran around the parking lot in front of the hotel. I was afraid she would get hit by a car and tried to corral her, but she was having none of it. Mom was inside and she was free. I kept easing closer, trying to grab an arm to lead her back to a safer place near the front door.

Suddenly, she flopped down on the driveway, and still laughing, lay flat down on the pavement, moving both arms and both legs back and forth. She was making "snow angels" on the concrete. Seeing my chance, I ran over and took her arm. I helped her up, and we walked back to the benches outside the hotel. She was giggling.

"Penny, let's sit here and wait for mom. She will be out in just a little bit."

I thought she would sit next to me, but she saw my brother on the opposite bench and ran over to him. She plopped herself down close to him, stuck her left thumb in her mouth, and snuggled up. I was thinking how comfortable she seemed with strangers, when suddenly she glanced up at my brother, reached out her right hand, and grabbed his crotch. He looked startled.

Thoughts raced through my mind. Maybe Alice was prostituting Penny. I quickly jumped up and ran over to her.

"No, Penny, come sit with me," I instructed as I took her arm and guided her back to where I was sitting.

Alice soon got checked in. We took Penny to her mom's room and left the pair at the hotel.

My curiosity got the best of me. Why was Penny on the street? Why were they begging? They both looked as if they had been homeless for a long time. The girl was obviously disabled and would qualify for government benefits. I assumed the mother was either mentally ill or substance addicted.

The next morning, I headed to the police station. I wanted to know the story of these two and see what was going on.

The first officer I spoke with directed me to another officer who "knew all about Penny and Alice." Officer Brenham was the "unofficial" go-to officer for this homeless pair. When I talked with him, I discovered this was not a new situation. They had been at that main intersection next to the interstate off and on for years. Sometimes they would leave for a few days, but then they would be back, begging again. He and other officers had been especially concerned about the girl. Some in the community even suspected sexual abuse. They believed the mom was tricking her out.

The police department had called Children's Services, but no one seemed to want to get involved. Officer Brenham told me the police department had fielded dozens of calls from concerned community members about Penny and her mom, but no one knew what to do. The agency they had contacted, whose job it was to care for kids such as Penny and investigate possible abuse, had failed repeatedly to act. I was appalled.

We have been conditioned to believe that if the state doesn't step in, nothing can be done about abuse or neglect. Somehow, our personal sense of responsibility remains dormant, even though our sympathies are aroused.

Of course there was something that could be done. We just had to figure out what that something was. First, we needed to get more information. Officer Brenham seemed hopeful after our conversation and said that he would give my contact info to anyone in the community who called him

about Penny. That's how it started.

Soon, I was receiving information from community members. Some had been trying to keep track of Penny for years. They all had stories of abuse, neglect, and a mentally unstable mother. I now knew more than enough to act, so I began by calling Children's Services. Yes, they knew about the young Down syndrome girl living on the street. No, they were not going to get involved.

Next, I went to the Down Syndrome Association and spoke with the director. She seemed sympathetic but was quick to remind me that getting involved to help this intellectually challenged girl with Down syndrome was not their job. Not mine either, I wanted to say. And what nonsense. Your organization is about support for those with Down syndrome and their families, I wanted to say. But I didn't. I thanked her and left, more than a little disgusted.

Meanwhile, the calls from the community kept coming in. Citizens told their personal stories of interactions with the pair, and a clear picture was beginning to emerge. These calls and e-mails were extremely helpful since we needed to know more about how Penny lived, and her mother refused to talk to anyone, except to ask for money. We needed to know if she was being cared for, where she slept, if she needed medical attention. I knew that many kids with Down syndrome had heart defects, vision and hearing problems, blood disorders, and hypothyroidism, as well as other conditions.

It was fall and the weather was getting cooler, especially at night. It would soon be winter, and I felt the clock ticking. Where did they go when it got too dark to beg? I had been told they slept under a nearby interstate at times, but I couldn't confirm it.

There were three community members who contacted me regularly. They were persistent in their calls, wanting to know what they could do for Penny. We decided to meet at a coffee shop, where we talked for a long time, pooling our information and brainstorming ideas.

We had nothing in common, really. One was a former flight attendant turned soccer mom, one was an aspiring singer-songwriter who had moved to the area from California, the third was a businessman from Australia, and then there was me. But we bonded quickly because we had the same goal: get Penny off the street and into a stable situation that provided for her needs.

We soon discovered that, contrary to what Alice had told us, Penny was not a child. Although she was only 4' 2" inches tall, she was almost twenty years old. Her feet and hands were tiny, and she wore a size 12 1/2 shoe. (That size usually fits a six- or seven-year-old girl.) Well, I thought, since she was over eighteen, Adult Protective Services could provide support for her. When I explained the situation and asked for them to investigate, the excuses began.

"Well, we've been called about them before. Several times." (But you didn't check into it?)

"I get off at 4:30 pm. I don't think I have time." (It's only 2:30 pm, but why can't you go in the morning?) "You know, the mother and daughter move around a lot. It's hard to know where to find them." (Not really, the local police department usually knows where they are.)

I got frustrated and decided to call another day and hopefully get someone more helpful. A few days later I called again and asked for a supervisor. I reexplained the situation.

Yes, he was familiar with the woman and daughter with Down syndrome living on the street.

They were hard to locate to investigate. (This time I was ready. I had called from my car across the street from where they were begging. Not today, I told him. I have my eyes on them right now.)

He hem-hawed around and giving no reason, refused to come out to talk to them. He also didn't say they would check up on them later. Nothing. I got nothing.

I was irate. As far as Penny was concerned, Children's Services, Adult Protective Services, and the Down Syndrome Association were useless. So I guess our little community group, the four of us, had to do this without them. I called another meeting at the coffee shop. I had an idea.

The first thing we needed to do was make sure we kept up with Penny's location. That meant one of us needed to have her in sight as much as possible. We communicated often with each other about sightings. We didn't want to lose track of her, but we had to be careful. If Alice knew what we were up to, there was a good chance she would take Penny and leave the state. (One of the local citizens told us this had happened before when concerned people started getting too close. Alice took Penny, left the state, and lived with an Amish community for a year before returning and resuming her life on the streets.)

We didn't need hearsay, we needed facts. We heard from people in the community that Alice had been offered jobs and housing multiple times, which she always refused. She wanted to live on the street. She wanted to beg. That was her choice.

But Penny had the mind of a child. She didn't choose to live that way, wondering where she would sleep, or when she would eat next. One of the things I had noticed was that Penny was thin. That was uncommon in people with Down syndrome. Later I found out that her mother restricted her food intake, left her hair long and scraggly, and purposely dressed her in clothes that didn't fit so she would garner more sympathy, resulting in more money. And it worked.

One of the police officers who had watched them for a long time estimated Alice made $30,000 to $40,000 annually in untaxed donations because of Penny. Kind, caring people were generous with food and money, and gave Penny clothes, toys, blankets, even a small bike. The problem was that these items were taken from her by Alice and returned to the store for cash. People who encountered them regularly figured this out and began cutting tags out of new clothing before they gave it to

Penny. That would ensure a store wouldn't accept the merchandise back and issue a refund. But Penny still didn't get to wear the clothes. They were placed in bags and put in the car. When Alice's van filled up, the items were placed in an old, broken-down car she owned. When that was stuffed full, she placed donated items in one of three storage units she had rented. She was a true hoarder.

Our community team spent weeks tracking down and talking to anyone who had had contact with this pair over the past several years, and a pattern emerged. Penny was definitely being exploited. She was made to sit by the side of the road or stand on a three-foot-wide concrete median with cars whizzing by on each side as her mother begged. We made notes of what we heard, and what we observed. We took photos. One team member made friends with them, buying them food, and taking them places when Alice's old car broke down. He took them out to eat for Christmas and bought presents for Penny. I didn't realize when we first began working together that he had a sister back in Australia who had Down syndrome. No wonder he had a special place in his heart for Penny.

We had gathered our information, so we executed part two of our plan. Find an attorney and petition the court for emergency conservatorship of Penny. We had our documented proof of abuse, and Officer Brenham agreed to testify on Penny's behalf. I would be the individual named as potential conservator, since I was familiar with state programs that could support Penny by renting her a home, providing staff, education, necessities, and medical care.

We found an attorney who did conservatorships for families of kids with intellectual disabilities and filed the petition. We were going to court.

Alice was furious. She showed up with Penny in tow, having gotten an attorney last minute to represent her. Officer Brenham was the primary witness, and Alice had the chance to defend herself against the accusations. This hearing was to determine if Penny needed to be removed immediately for her health and safety. The judge decided there was enough evidence against Alice that he ordered Penny to be placed under my care temporarily until the situation could be further investigated. In the meantime, Alice would be allowed to have supervised visits with Penny, and a guardian ad litem would be appointed to represent Penny's best interests by gathering and presenting facts for the court to consider. After all the facts were weighed, the judge would then decide on more permanent guardianship.

We were joined in the courtroom by a new team member who offered to use her small agency to provide Penney's daily care if the judge approved. She was a single mom with a big heart and a special love for those with intellectual disabilities. She had overcome many obstacles to be able to build her own business caring for adults with special needs. She was a godsend.

After hearing from everyone involved, the judge made his decision. Penny would not be leaving with her mother. She would be placed under my temporary conservatorship until further investigation could be carried out.

The tension in the courtroom was palatable. The judge instructed Alice to stay behind, giving us time to collect Penny and leave the courthouse. It was now winter, and as we walked out into the cold night air, I was conscious of the fact that Penny had on a dirty cotton t-shirt and a long cotton skirt about four sizes too large. It was safety-pinned at the waist to keep it from falling off her small body. She had no coat, no sweater, no cap or gloves, and thin canvas shoes with no socks. Soon she would be warm, though. I had bought winter outerwear and it was waiting in my car in case the judge approved the emergency petition.

The first place we went was to a nearby Shoney's. I knew Penny would be hungry. She asked for chicken and fries; at least that's what we thought she said. One of the things she would need was speech therapy. I made a mental note.

I thought Penny would be distressed at being separated from her mother, but she didn't appear agitated or perturbed in any way. She acted as if being taken from her mother in a courtroom by total strangers was perfectly normal. Over the course of the next several months, I kept watching for a separation reaction of some sort. Depression, crying, throwing fits, anxiety; something to show the depth of the bond between her and her mom. It never came.

CHAPTER 26

For the Love of Penny

The full story of Penny and Alice is for another time. I have included parts of it in this book as an example of what a community, ordinary citizens, can do to assist the vulnerable if they are committed and focused.

I visited Rugby, Tennessee, several years ago and was impressed by this quote by Thomas Hughes in 1880. His goal was to establish a Utopian community free of the rigid class distinctions that he experienced in England. It would be focused on agriculture but have a culturally refined atmosphere. He took the step, and Rugby, Tennessee, came into existence. It was a cooperative community that grew to have 600 to 700 Victorian buildings, including a theater and a fabulous library that still stands today. But he and his cofounders were not naive. They knew what they were up against.

"Pausing a moment to look on before

Seeing the goal as it shines more and more

Fearing defeat, yet longing to win

Trembling and wavering, thus we begin."

Anytime we step out of our comfort zones to tackle something new, to fulfill a dream, to put ourselves at risk, to chart new territory we know we may fail. There may be consequences, good and bad, we never dreamed of. That's life.

Although I expected some of the less than desirable consequences of getting Penny off the streets, I was also blindsided by some of them. I didn't expect legal battles to continue for four years. I didn't expect to have a lawsuit filed against me personally, as well as twenty-one other defendants including the governor, the state attorney general, and many others. I didn't expect the judge who ruled in the case to receive a bomb threat. I didn't expect Penny's case to become a "cause celebre" in the Internet world against conservatorship in general. I didn't expect the media coverage or that certain homeless "advocates" would make it their personal goal to reunite Penny with her mother and let them continue living on the street. I didn't expect a kidnapping plot. There were myriads of things I never expected.

My strong belief is that consequences should not determine our actions. Right is right regardless of what occurs after an action is taken. But not all situations result in a happy outcome. Thankfully, Penny had a heartwarming ending to her story.

After leaving the restaurant I took Penny home with me. I checked her head for lice, washed her hair, and instructed her to take a bath. She dressed herself in brand new, pretty pajamas, brushed her teeth, and then looked at herself in the mirror, smiling broadly. With her right hand she made a circular motion in front of her face. It was one of the few signs I knew.

"Yes," I said, meeting her eyes in the mirror. "Penny is beautiful."

She ran, jumped in bed, and placed her thumb in her mouth. She fell asleep quickly.

Suddenly, I felt the staggering weight of the responsibility I had just assumed. Penny was neither my client nor my child. She had a mother, yet the court appointed *me* to be responsible for her health, her safety, her life. I suddenly became conscious of the fact that I was in brand new territory, way out of my comfort zone. Reaching over, I gently stroked her cheek. She looked so vulnerable, so trusting, as she slept.

I knew the next day and the next and the next would be full of discovery and getting Penny settled in her new home. There would be legal battles—Alice would never give up her daughter without a fight—and all kinds of problems to address that we had not even had time to consider.

She would need a medical and dental examination. We would need to set up regular, supervised visitation with her mother. She needed everything: clothes, toys, books, toiletries.

She would need therapy: speech, behavioral, perhaps nutritional. We would need to apply for social security. She would need furniture, bedding, linens, dishes. Staff would need to be hired to supervise and transport her. She was twenty; the state provided schooling until she reached twenty-one, so she would need to complete her education. There was much to do.

Penny's newest team member took care of most of the physical things Penny needed and hired staff to care for her. I focused more on legal issues, and Penny's court-ordered visitation with Alice. The visits did not go well. Most were held in public places like a large room in a local library, but the library asked us to cease our visits after Alice kept bringing strangers to confront us, causing a stir. At times, we had to have paid security at the visits. We briefly tried meeting at Penny's new home, but after one visit, staff found bedbugs so Alice was not allowed back. We had to keep finding new locations for the visits.

Alice wanted a show and brought unapproved people with her many times to see Penny. She would pretend these people were Penny's friends, but Penny didn't know them. She got a photographer to sneak and take photos through windows. She did not like the fact that Penny looked and dressed differently and wanted the photos as evidence to show the court that we were changing her. She hated Penny's wonderful staff; actually, she hated anyone who supported Penny. Penny was her property and meal ticket. And she had lost her to strangers. We were the bad guys.

For the first time in her life, Penny was allowed to choose what she wore and what she ate. She wanted to get her hair cut, so one of the team took her to a beauty salon where she chose a shoulder-length cut. She wanted her nails polished, so she got her nails done. She was living her own life. Interestingly, Penny never acted like she missed her mom, but she seemed to enjoy the weekly visits with her. I realized she was conflicted, though, when after a visit with Alice, she would come to me, sign "Mama bad," and watch for my reaction.

"Yes," I would say, "Mama bad. But you love your mama and that's ok. You can have a good visit with Mama and then go back to Penny's house."

She would sign, "I love you," and I would sign back to her the same. Then she would look up at me, smile, and take my hand. Penny knew she was safe, and she was going home. *Her* home.

CHAPTER 27

Brokenness

One of the terms mental health workers are encouraged not to use is "broken." For example, a person, regardless of issues, is not "broken" so they can't be "fixed." I think I understand the reasoning behind the desire to remove the word from our vocabulary, but I beg to disagree. While there are times the concept is true, there are also times when situations and people *are* broken. Acknowledgment of this fact can often lead to healing and restoration.

I have worked with many clients who were born with Down syndrome. They are not broken, they simply have an additional chromosome. They are generally happy and loving, although they experience the full range of human emotions just like everyone else. The additional chromosome places them in the category of being intellectually challenged, but most live happy and fulfilling lives. An abstract found in the *American*

Journal of Medical Genetics (Published 2011, Part A/Volume 155, Issue 10) illustrates this well.

The authors, Skoto, Levine, and Goldstein, asked a group of 284 people with Down Syndrome, age twelve and older, several questions about themselves. Among those surveyed, the average age of the respondents was twenty-three years old. The results were enlightening: 99 percent indicated they were happy with their lives, 97 percent liked who they were, and 96 percent liked how they looked.

When you consider the population who are considered normal, I doubt you can find a study anywhere that will give you these types of happiness numbers. It is remarkable feedback from a group of people whom we might assume had much to be unhappy about. I do not consider them to be broken and in need of fixing.

But there is another group of people with issues and disorders that affect everything they do and keep them from having a good quality of life. Someone who is bipolar; or schizophrenic; or suffers from post-traumatic stress disorder; or suffers from crippling anxiety or depression; or addiction; or a thousand other issues are in a broken state; they are not whole. They can be helped by medication, therapies, counseling, and other types of supports. Some can be fixed, although honesty demands that I admit some disorders can only be *managed.* But relationships, job opportunities, day-to-day living can be greatly improved. They can be productive and happy.

In many ways, this is a broken world. You only have to follow the news for one cycle to see and feel that truth. But hope, blessed hope, keeps us moving forward. As social workers, we well know we cannot fix the whole world. But on a good day, we can fix little pieces of it and know we have made a small difference. That's more than many people ever have the opportunity to do.

The beauty of this irritating, satisfying, unpredictable profession is that it changes us. We hope, we pray, we *expect* to see changes and success in those we work with and for. Sometimes, we get to see and experience these changes in others; sometimes we don't. But every act of service, every task we perform causes a change in *us*.

The more I see firsthand the struggles and tragedies of those I work with, the more I realize that I need them as much, maybe more, than they need me. That was a gradual yet startling revelation. I need them.

Social work will never make you wealthy. The nonprofits or state agencies either don't have the money to pay what is deserved or undervalue the contribution social workers make to society. Just like with first responders, the pay is not commensurate with the services provided. It is also not commensurate with the risks taken. But another reason social workers will never be wealthy is because much of what is made will go to those served.

Our position puts us in the middle of a sea of need. It surrounds us. Sometimes the need is so great it takes your breath away, and it cannot be filled. But you do what you can.

You buy a mattress for the child sleeping on a hard floor. You buy groceries, and groceries, and more groceries because that 250-pound, 6' 3" young man who is intellectually challenged cannot live on $36 of food stamps a month. You utilize social services and are grateful for them, but too many people fall through the cracks and do not qualify for one reason or another. Perhaps they cannot take time off from their minimum wage job to spend half a day in line to apply for help, only to find out they lack one document they need and must reset an appointment for a month later. But their employer says if they take off again, he will fire them. Or perhaps that mother of four, who cleans houses while trying to care for her terminally husband who lies dying at home, has no transportation or extra money for Uber. She can't even speak our language yet, but you can see pure need in her eyes.

You beg from friends. You solicit donations from businesses. But at the end of the day, most of it comes out of your pocket. Because each need has a face and a name. There is no anonymity here. You see each person clearly.

Not all needs can be met. And although you know this acutely, you will still take those fails to heart and carry them with you. It is a heavy burden to bear, knowing that regardless of how much you help or give, it is never, ever enough. This is not a job you can complete and then move on. It becomes part of who you are. It binds to your heart.

If you find yourself not caring enough and blocking out cries for help, if you are working only for the salary, it is time for you to stop. If you are a social worker, this is my advice to you: either take a break until you are no longer numb to the pain around you or turn in your social worker badge and go do something else. You will do more harm than good. Treat your profession like the valuable service it is. Respect it.

I hope the honesty of this book doesn't scare anyone away who has considered becoming a social worker. There is no better occupation. But new workers need to go into the field with open eyes, and full commitment. They need to understand and be willing to take the risks involved. In my many years working in both rural and urban environments, I have been blessed. By the Lord's good grace, I have never been badly hurt. Most people I encounter are either supportive or indifferent to actions I may take. But I have had to develop a tough skin. At times, I have upset many people: family members of clients, employees and/or directors of governmental agencies, doctors, police officers, community organizations, even other social workers. And of course, clients themselves. I have been threatened, followed, and slandered on Internet podcasts. I have been publicly attacked in a newspaper. I have been ignored by social service agencies I called on for help. I have been sued and have had my personal life scrutinized in open court. I have been cursed more times than I can remember. I have been accused of doing what I do for the money. These were done not by clients but by those who are supposed to have the best interests of our vulnerable population at heart.

By clients the risks were more physical. I have been spat on, kicked, scratched and shoved. One punch delivered a black eye. I had a knife pulled on me, and another time a man held a brick to my head and threatened to bash it in. When I worked in a public institution, two of the clients waited behind my car after dark intending to rape me. But they had bragged about it, and someone snitched on them. (I was escorted out of my workplace after dark, and they quickly ran off.) I have been stalked, screamed at, threatened, and called vulgar names. This is just the reality of field work in the mental health field.

But I have also worked with many wonderful, salt-of-the-earth people who volunteer time and money, and more time and more money, to those who need help. Professionals, ordinary citizens, police officers, lawyers, court officials, private business owners; I couldn't begin to name them all.

Remember Penny's story? Different taxpayer supported social service departments were aware of her plight and had failed her, over and over, for *seventeen years.* But the community stepped in. What the state agencies would not do over almost two decades, this small group of ordinary citizens accomplished in just a few short months. They did the leg work and spent an untold number of hours on her behalf. They succeeded because they persisted.

I have a small art plaque on my desk designed by Leigh Stanley. On it is a sketch of a skinny young girl in a t-shirt and flip flops. She is on her bike, legs sticking out to the sides away from the pedals. As she coasts, she looks carefree and untroubled. It makes me smile.

But it is the words that I like most.

"I am fairly certain that given a cape and a nice tiara, I could save the world."

It is a good tongue-in-cheek definition of the heart of a social worker.

Epilogue

Here is where I get to pontificate.

Character counts. If you are going to guide or influence people you work with, if you really want to make a difference, be a role model. Trust is critical to success. If you don't want to be lied to, don't lie. If you don't want to be threatened or` cursed, don't threaten or curse. Be as nonjudgmental as you realistically can be. Just because someone is intellectually challenged or has a mental disorder doesn't mean you can skimp on human kindness.

Listen.

Be direct, but kind.

Use humor whenever possible.

Show respect.

Be compassionate.

Be thick-skinned.

Focus on your goals and don't let minor things distract you.

Pick your battles.

Pick your battles.

Pick your battles.

Be professional.

Stay in control of your emotions, especially when everyone else is falling apart.

Give hope.

Give second chances.

Have I mentioned you should pick your battles?

In Rudyard Kipling's poem titled *If*, he tells his son how to become a man. One of the lines states

If you can keep your head when all about you
are losing theirs and blaming it on you . . .

This, to me, is the essence of being a social worker. The work is usually messy, and we are dealing with people in crisis. Let's be honest, that's not when we show ourselves in the best light. All our human emotions come into play, often several at a time. Anger, fear, and resentment often show up together. Despair, anxiety, and fear can be comrades. Sadness, shame, guilt, embarrassment, confusion, anxiety. Any of these negative emotions can be present in the same person at the same time. In crisis, we don't see as many of the positive emotions, but they can be present as well and complicate the mix. For example, the same client who is furious one day can show gratitude the next time you see him. We often observe strength, endurance, and resilience mixed in with negative emotions.

The challenge for any good citizen, any decent human being, is to rise above the fray of human emotions; be kind, be compassionate, but stay focused on the outcome you hope to achieve. And stay optimistic. You can't pass on hope if you don't have it yourself. Share your faith generously, but be stingy with your doubts.

Realize that every person and situation of which you are part will teach you something. Your goal is to help, to facilitate, to change lives. But here is an absolute truth: whether or not you are able to improve the person's circumstances, or make even a small difference in their lives, *you* will change. And that change, that experience, not only pushes you toward personal growth but better equips you to assist the next person. Bad experiences and failures can be the best teachers.

Take nothing personally. This is a hard one, especially if you are being cussed at, threatened, called vulgar names, being spit on, whatever. There is a saying I came across that has helped me a lot.

"When you finally learn that a person's behavior has more to do with their internal struggle than it has with you, you learn grace" (attributed to Allison Aars).

Bad behavior—whether in a person with a developmental disability, or a mental disorder, or exhibited by someone with neither—says more about them than it does about you. Don't carry grudges, don't let personal affronts seep into your soul. You are responsible for how you respond, not for what they do. Acting badly is almost always a choice. And choices have consequences.

Be open minded and willing to listen. Take criticism, whether deserved or not. Experienced workers gave me invaluable advice, but I didn't always listen, because I thought I knew more than I did. What I actually had was zeal without knowledge. But time and experience are great teachers. Nothing, nothing, nothing takes the place of field work. Create relationships with real people with real problems. And listen to those who have been there, done that.

Never show fear. Fear is contagious and it helps few situations. Show calm on your face and in your speech and body as much as you can. We are all afraid of something; most of us have a list of somethings. But fear leads to anxiety. and anxiety cycles back to fear. and we are caught in an endless loop that focuses on our feelings over our predicament and other people's needs. In crisis, we are called to be the voice of calm, the voice of reason. Stay the chaos.

I have many more stories. I could tell you about Liz, the woman with no teeth whom we called "The Spitter" because she worked many years to turn her spit into a weapon. I could tell you about Lenny who, even with my twenty years plus of social work experience, conned me good. This cowboy-hat wearing, guitar strumming, twenty-something year old country guy who was intellectually challenged convinced me he once played in front of 10,000 screaming fans. I still can't explain how I bought into *that* fantasy.

I could tell you about Charisse, who would holler, "Police! Help!" on Halloween when she wanted more candy, getting attention from passersby. I have many stories left to tell. And I plan to accumulate them until I can no longer work.

My name is Belinda, and I am still a social worker.

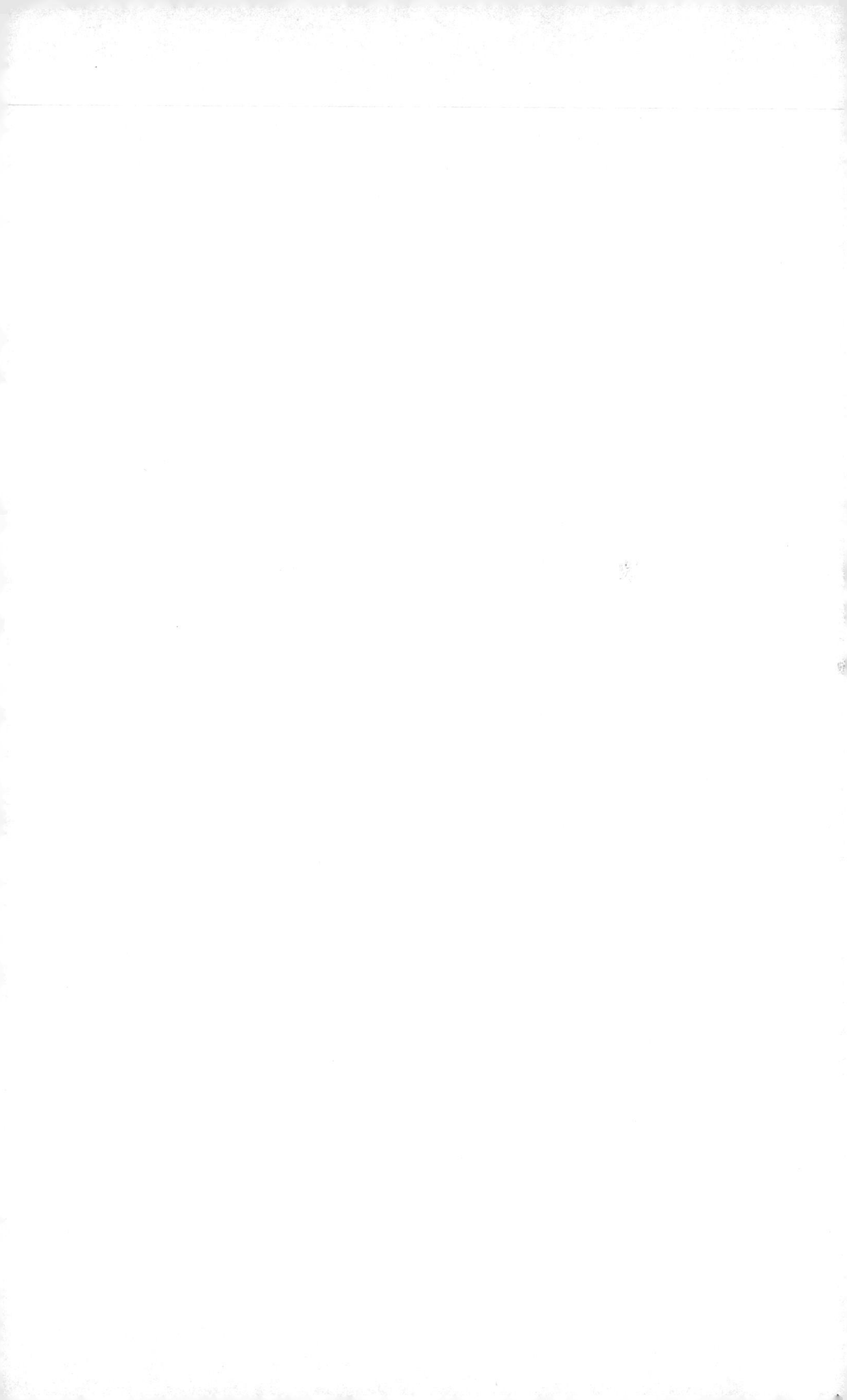

Made in the USA
Monee, IL
22 December 2023

50408971R00185